THE PEACH

THE PEACH

A Memoir of Trauma, Survival, and Forgiveness

Melissa H. Cronin

Mnemosyne Books

Praise for The Peach

"Melissa Cronin was a highly skilled NICU nurse, an accomplished athlete who climbed mountains and was in peak physical condition when she was blindsided at a farmer's market by an out-of-control driver who killed ten people. Melissa woke up two days later in a hospital, her life changed forever. *The Peach* is a remarkable story of sudden violence and loss, the long road to recovery, and the ultimate redemptive power of forgiveness, written in luminous prose with an honesty that is gripping and raw, interspersed with welcome flashes of wit and humor."

—Marianne Leone
Author of *Jesse: A Mother's Story* and *Five Dog Epiphany*

"With horrendous trauma, survival and healing are often precarious and not always achieved. Melissa Cronin writes about her near-death experience at the 2003 Santa Monica Farmer's Market, with heart-wrenching honesty and clarity. Once started, I found *The Peach* difficult to put down. As a psychotherapist, I retired after over 30 years of treating veterans, sexual trauma victims, and survivors of a variety of human horrors with Post-Traumatic Stress Disorder. This book gives hope to those who have also suffered great tragedy and pain. Healing is indeed possible with the right treatment, support, time, and patience."

— Madeleine Tobias, MS RN CS (retired),
Author of *God, Dogs, and UFOs, a memoir.*

"It stands as a reminder that there are still those rare human beings who choose to turn their back on the dark and walk bravely toward the light."

— Mira Bartok
Author of *The New York Times* best-selling memoir, *The Memory Palace.*

"Every traumatic brain injury is unique, yet Melissa Cronin captures the universal core of that kaleidoscopic experience; world-shattering and profoundly transformational at the same time."

—Carolyn Roy-Bornstein
Author of *Crash: A Mother, a Son, and the Journey from Grief to Gratitude.*

Published by
MNEMOSYNE BOOKS
An Imprint of
SAINT JULIAN PRESS, Inc.
2053 Cortlandt, Suite 200
Houston, Texas 77008
www.saintjulianpress.org

This memoir is based on the author's
recollections of events and experiences.
Certain names and identifying details have been
changed to protect the privacy of persons.

Print ISBN-13: 978-1-955194-56-3
eBook ISBN-13: 978-1-955194-57-0
Library of Congress Control Number: 2026944217

Cover Image:
Yuri Gurevich/Shutterstock.com
Book Design:
Smythtype Design

for John

Contents

Part III

While conversations have been reconstructed to the best of my recollection, all events depicted in this book are based on my memories, extensive research into personal journals, archival records, public records, and contemporaneous accounts.

Some names have been changed to maintain the anonymity of certain individuals.

THE PEACH

Prelude

I dig my nails into my thigh, scrape the center of the raw moon-shaped scar. The itch won't let up. My nail catches on something hard and sharp. A splinter? I tweeze it out. A sliver of glass, the size of a fingernail tip. My leg itches all afternoon and evening, into the next day. For several days, the itch wakes me during the night.

Years later, my leg still itches. The itch connects me to the day my moon scar was born. The day ten people died. I am one of the others, the ones who did not die. But what most people might not understand is that there is a kind of death that goes along with surviving. A part of us is forever changed. There is no going back to the before.

Each time I run my fingers over the spot with the itch, I am spirited back to the day it was engraved upon me, and I am once again flooded with fear, back among those who have seen death up close, replaying it over and over, in the form of our stories. Today, my scars are my story—of a woman who was about to take a bite of a perfect peach on a beautiful summer afternoon.

More than ever before, motor vehicles are being used—both intentionally and unintentionally—as weapons of mass destruction. "Mass" as in the numbers of lives they extinguish and the massive blow they inflict upon survivors and families of the dead. Even your vehicle and mine can be transformed into engines of destruction in a matter of seconds, making us all vulnerable in ways we've hardly contemplated before.

Part I

Chapter 1

I walk along Arizona Avenue in Santa Monica, my sneakers making that squish, squish sound of synthetic rubber against pavement. Apricots, plums, and pears lie in long orderly rows. They all look so yummy. I can't make up my mind which vendor to stop at first. The air is gauzy. Parasols, towering over the marketplace like giant sunflowers, protect shoppers from the summer sun. Voices collide. "*Tres por un dólar.*" "I'll take a dozen." "*Pruebe una muestra.*" A little girl skips after seagulls waddling across wet mirages on the pavement. A mother leans on the handles of a stroller that holds her infant son. A father grips the hand of his preschool-age daughter.

I glance at my wristwatch. It's 1:43 p.m. The Santa Monica Farmers' Market closes at 2 p.m. People scurry past me in search of the last berries, tomatoes, artisan cheeses, and tropical fruits. At the intersection of Arizona Avenue and the Third Street Promenade, making my way toward Second Street, I pass a snoring homeless man, an empty amber bottle at his side. I continue walking. I'm thirsty and hungry.

Through the crowd of shoppers and maze of reds, greens, and purples, I spot a pyramid of peaches that makes my mouth water. Every summer gifts you with at least one juicy peach, one that rewards you with peach sweetness. I walk to the other side of Arizona Avenue and carefully pick up a perfectly plump one. I roll it in my hand, its reddish-hued skin warmed by the afternoon sun, its downy fuzz tickling my fingers. I bring the peach to my nose. It smells like orchard sugar. I can't wait to take the first bite—the squirt, the pulp, the tang.

That's when I hear the *pop*. And the peach flies out of my hand.

I do not remember a Buick sedan heading toward me as its eighty-six-year-old driver pressed his foot to the accelerator, believing he was pressing the brake.

I do not remember the Buick striking bodies. *Boom, boom, boom.*

I do not remember the bumper catching a little girl and dragging her away. Nor do I remember another child lying in the street covered in blood, his mother screaming, "My baby, my baby!"

I do not remember tables toppling, umbrellas snapping, boxes collapsing.

I do not remember the Buick racing two-and-a-half blocks before coming to a stop, people splayed on its hood and windshield.

I do not remember a woman trapped beneath the car, or bystanders scrambling to lift it off her.

I do not remember asking a woman who knelt by my side as I lay on the ground groaning, "Where is the ambulance? Where is the ambulance?"

I do not remember firefighters carrying me on a backboard to a helicopter two blocks away, lifting me into the chopper, and flying me from Santa Monica, eastward, to Los Angeles General Medical Center.

I do not remember the blades spinning fast, slicing dense air. *Whop, whop, whop.*

What I do remember: lying on a stretcher in the emergency room, surrounded by too much white, white stinging my eyes. Burning-cold air floating into my lungs. Pain rising from my throat. I couldn't hear my own screams, as if someone had filled my ears with sawdust.

I remember not being able to turn my head, and thinking, *I'm in a neck brace.* Then a face looking down at me: a balding man with bushy eyebrows.

He placed his strong hand on my limp arm, and said, "You've been in an accident."

I remember stethoscopes swaying around necks. Dings and beeps. Mechanical voices talking from the ceiling. A woman leaning over me, the even ends of her long black hair brushing against my hand. Her lips, smeared berry red, moving fast, like she had something urgent to tell me. I couldn't hear her. She disappeared.

I remember a petite girl with protruding eyes and wild curls pushing me into a cold machine, a CAT scan. Her round eyes and face zoomed farther and farther out of focus. Then she was gone, as suddenly as the red-lipped woman.

I remember the man with the bushy eyebrows saying something about my spleen "bleeding."

"We need to take you to the operating room."

I remember asking, "Am I going to make it?"

And the man assuring me, "We're going to take care of you."

I remember someone handing me a pen, and guiding it to a black line at the bottom of a yellow form, so I could sign my name, giving surgeons permission to remove my ruptured spleen. My arm was heavy, as if I was holding a gallon of water. I felt disconnected from my physical body, from the hand dragging the pen across the page. It took several seconds before I managed to sign my name: a large M followed by a series of squiggles, like a fading waveform on a cardiac monitor.

While doctors and nurses at LA General worked to save my life, doctors and nurses at other hospitals worked to treat and save the lives of as many as seventy-two others, all struck down by the same red Buick.

Chapter 2

Seven-month-old Brandon David Esfahani was bleeding from his ears when he arrived in the emergency room at UCLA Medical Center in Santa Monica. Nurses frantically cut off his gray-green pajamas to check for other injuries.

Fifty-year-old Kevin McCarthy, bleeding profusely from several places, arrived at Saint John's Health Center in Santa Monica. For more than five hours, doctors and nurses infused Kevin with large volumes of donated blood.

Eighty-nine-year-old Shamsi Khani, the oldest survivor, arrived at UCLA's emergency room unconscious. She sustained a ruptured temporal artery, and her right ear was sliced in half. Along with hip and leg fractures, her neck was broken. A doctor told her family she had a ninety percent chance of being paralyzed.

Twenty-five-year-old Jenna Edwards was treated at UCLA Medical Center for leg, back, and neck injuries.

Forty-seven-year-old Sandra Bacall suffered from a fractured and dislocated left shoulder. She also had multiple lacerations and an injured left foot.

Sixty-year-old Ilona Lettrich was treated for injuries to her ankles, arms, and ribs. Three of her fingers were almost severed.

Sixty-one-year-old Bartley Bard was flown by helicopter to a nearby trauma center with severe head injuries. He was admitted to the intensive care unit in critical condition, then taken to the operating room for brain surgery.

The eighty-six-year-old driver was taken to UCLA Medical Center, examined by doctors, then released to speak with the Santa Monica police. He sustained no physical injuries.

Chapter 3

During the first three days after surgery, I remain heavily sedated. Yellow-and-red strobe lights stream toward me through a window, the side-to-side rocking motion blurring the colors orange. I'm being transferred by ambulance to a different campus of LA General. My mother appears next to me: her brown bob, her russet eyes, her washed-out face. Later, she appears again, in a chair at the foot of my hospital bed, her brow creased as she stares at me, like a first-time mother watching over her bruised newborn. The room turns black as a midnight lake.

A white-coated physician stands by my bedside. I see him through what looks like a curved mirror, making him appear distorted, his arms and legs too long for his stout body.

"Your foot," he says. "Broken…cast." He sounds as if he is speaking under water.

I try to speak, but all that comes out is a throaty moan and my eyes close. It is dark again. When I wake, I try to lift my leg, but it's weighed down by something solid: a hard cast, from foot to knee.

A nurse leaning over me, her voice like pieces of Styrofoam rubbing together, directing me to press a red button on a remote control to deliver extra doses of morphine.

"It'll help you," she says.

I'm afraid of the morphine, afraid of being driven into a distant sphere by my own hand, now numb and unreliable, or by someone else's hand. It doesn't comfort me that I am a neonatal intensive care nurse and have experienced others in a medical crisis—I injected hundreds of babies with narcotics, and they kept breathing. It doesn't comfort me that the morphine control device has a built-in safety mechanism, making it impossible to overdose.

I shake my head at the nurse. She pushes the button for me. Again, my eyes close. I feel nothing. My fear falls asleep.

Chapter 4

The summer of 2003 was the summer I chose to run away, far from the man with whom I spent seven years too long. I was thirty-six and finally decided I needed to move on with my life. I started with a trip to Santa Monica, where my sister lived. After the six-hour flight from Vermont, I looked forward to a week of sea-spritzed breezes, away from my long shifts in the NICU.

—

I check into my hotel room and wander down to the Santa Monica Farmers' Market.

My body rockets into the air and slams against the pavement, the impact jarring my brain, rupturing my spleen, fracturing my pelvis, sacrum, multiple ribs, left foot, and tearing off the bony projections from my lumbar spine. Everything comes to a screeching halt, then spins in reverse.

I do not die.

Why do I not die?

Brandon David Esfahani, 7 months

Cindy Palacios Valladares, 3

Gloria Gonzalez, 35

Diana Gong McCarthy, 41

Lynne Weaver, 47

Theresa Breglia, 50

Kevin McCarthy, 50

Leroy Lattier, 55

Molok Ghoulian Nabatian, 63

Movsha Hoffman, 78

All ten of those individuals perish. I lie in a hospital bed, tethered to monitors and IVs, yet still alive.

Chapter 5

On the afternoon of July 15, just hours before my flight landed in California, I went for a long run on Vermont back country roads. Wearing broken-in sneakers that were molded to my feet, I ran and ran, my feet rising and falling, as though they possessed their own consciousness. I ran despite the pain—a bloody toe, a stiff knee, shin splints. I ran in the rain, in the snow, or in fifteen-degree weather with a bandana lightly wrapped around my mouth and nose to protect my lungs from the frigid air. I ran after working twelve-hour shifts, my consciousness floating along above my feet on a string tied to my laces. I trusted my autopilot feet to carry me home.

Since my junior year in high school, I embraced almost any kind of exercise, because it burned calories. I lost nearly forty pounds during my senior year and was diagnosed with anorexia nervosa. For people with anorexia, no amount of thinness is enough. For perfectionists, no amount of success is enough, so we tend to believe we're never good enough, and continuously punish ourselves for it. After years of therapy, I managed to maintain a healthy weight, and punished myself in less life-threatening ways, but ways that still put me at risk.

The summer before the accident, I joined two friends on the eight-and-a-half-mile climb up Mount Washington. For the first two miles, we trekked along smooth, wide trails, gradually making our way through the forest of hardwood, spruce, and fir. As we gained elevation into the subalpine zone, the trees became smaller, and we picked our way around gnarled and twisted krummholz vegetation. From there the trail grew steeper and rockier. I had to use my hands to clamber ahead. There are places in the world where we lose our advantage as a bipedal species, and this was surely one of them. After several minutes, I stopped to look behind me. And froze. The trail I had so slowly climbed would take more than courage to trek back down. I saw no real trail but a half-mile of scree, thousands and thousands of gray rocks. I scoured for something that would stop me from a fall to my death if I slipped.

"It's a little unnerving, isn't it?" one of my climbing mates asked. I nodded, but it was a lot unnerving. My gut was in free-fall and I thought I might actually shit my pants. I wanted to cry, to blurt out that I had made a moronic mistake by agreeing to go on the hike. But I was ashamed to reveal how terrified I was. I considered staying right there, with my fingernails clawed into a pocket of dirt until a search and rescue team unhinged me from this merciless mountain. I breathed and broke through the panic. I was in a battle of fear versus shame. With my eyes trained on what lay ahead of me—another four miles of rock-heavy terrain—I carefully reached for a rock, wiggling it to make sure it was secure enough to hold me, grabbed onto it and heaved myself upward. That's how I continued for the rest of the four miles: right hand reaching for a rock, right foot stepping up onto a rock. Left hand reaching. Left foot stepping.

Black flies started swarming around us. They flew into my ears, my mouth, my eyes. We had to keep moving. I scrambled ahead without looking back, stopping only for a sip of water from my CamelBak, and to wipe sweat from my hands on the bandana tied to my belt. My foot slipped. I shrieked in terror. My breath stopped. Seconds passed while I listened to the scree raining three thousand feet below me. I forced a breath sharply through my nose to blow away the flies, and inhaled, reaching for the next steady rock. I kept quiet during the rest of the hike. I needed to concentrate, to hear the voice inside my head. *You'll make it to the top. You're almost there. Take a step, another one. There you go. Don't you dare fucking quit.*

As I advanced upward, the sun climbed with me. I had never felt so near to this luminous body, its halo shimmering like a fiery white diamond. I climbed faster, reached higher, as if I could find the sun, touch it, step into its yellow glow. Finally, I reached a place where the scree disappeared, lifted my foot, then the other, planted both feet on hard, compact rock. Fireworks detonated inside of me, and my entire body trembled, relieved of the fear of falling headlong to my death, and awed that I had done it. I had climbed more than four thousand feet to the summit, the highest peak in the White Mountains of New Hampshire. Good enough for a flawed perfectionist. I was truly alive.

Chapter 6

My coworkers from the NICU send me a Vermont Teddy Bear. It's a hiker bear, outfitted in a red nylon backpack and hiking boots. Each time I wake in my hospital bed at LA General, I reach out to rub my hand along its golden-wheat furred belly—my Buddha bear—and I am back to those triumphant moments on Mount Washington.

My fiddle sits near the bed in its case, propped up so I can see it. I brought it with me to California so I wouldn't miss a day of practice while on vacation. Another toy in my bag of obsessions, the fiddle brings me back to sweeter days when I was excited to be with the friends I made while exploring Irish music. In June, three weeks before my fateful trip to California, Katrina, a new Irish fiddler friend, invited me to hear her band Trinity perform their upcoming gig.

"Maybe you can get up on stage with us sometime and play a few tunes," she said. I was bug-eyed thrilled at the idea, but also petrified. I had been playing Irish music for less than a year and had performed for only two people: my instructor and me.

On a hot evening I found myself in a pub, watching the trio perform to a crowd of regulars. During Trinity's break, I talked with Katrina and John, one of her band mates, on the front porch of the pub. The evening air was sticky. "I don't know how you guys do it," I said. "Get up there on stage? I'm not sure I could do that."

"I'm actually not a musician, and I get away with it," John said. "I'm more of an entertainer, having fun with the crowd between songs, telling jokes and Irish stories, raising pints."

I assumed "pint" meant a pint of Guinness, since he was holding a full one, and raised the glass as he spoke, affecting an Irish brogue. He was also wearing a t-shirt embroidered with a Guinness logo.

As he sipped the foam from the rim of the glass, then licked his lips clean, John eyed me in my spaghetti-strapped sundress. I glanced down at my feet, tripped sideways by such a look. I judged him to be much older than me, with his salt-and-pepper hair. And it had been two months since ending a seven-year relationship. I had promised myself I'd stay single for a while.

"Katrina tells me you're interested in getting out to play your fiddle," John said. "You should come to the open session I run up in Burlington. Every Wednesday I'm there. Seven o'clock."

"Sure," I said, convulsing from my fingers to my toes.

What the fuck did I just sign up for? I chided myself. *Melissa, you can't even keep time when playing your fiddle.*

Screw that. So what if I was still a novice? I'd have the chance to perform with "real" musicians. But I had other things going on: work, painting my apartment, mountain biking and hiking with friends. And preparing for my trip to California.

On July 10, after John sent me an email reminding me of the sessions, I responded. "When I get back from my trip, I'd love to join you."

Chapter 7

I'm an infant again. My mother feeds me Jell-O from a plastic spoon, my re-introduction to food five days after the accident. Slowly, she lifts the wiggly substance toward my mouth and gently pushes it between my chapped lips, shocking my taste buds.

"Yuck." I spit the tart blob back into the spoon.

"What's wrong with lemon?" she asks. "I thought you'd like it." She spoons out a new dose of Jell-O and tastes it. "This is actually pretty good."

There is nothing wrong with lemon, except I don't like it, never liked it as a child. But, yes, I'm sure it's pretty good—in my mother's world.

A nurse wanders into my room, interrupting my lemon delight. "I bet you'll be glad to know it's time to toss that in the trash," she says, pointing to the urinary catheter hanging from me like a long strand of undercooked linguine. She doesn't even have to ask me to spread my legs. "Ready?" she says, holding the catheter. "Here we go." One swift pull, then a hot sting straight through the bladder. It spasms, and there is no stopping it.

"I have to pee," I say. My mother springs up from her chair opposite the bed. As I reach for the side rail with both hands, she guides my stiff body to the right, releasing a hint of her thyme-scented soap. She slides one edge of the plastic bedpan by my side and rolls me onto my back. I squirm, searching for the most comfortable position, the sharp corners of the pan stabbing my thighs. I pee, keep peeing. The urine is hot and smells like ammonia.

"Mom, can you help me? I can't reach." My neck and arms won't move. They're rigid, like plywood.

"Of course, I can help."

She rolls me onto my side and wipes me dry.

Ten minutes later: "Mom. Sorry. I need to go again."

Again, my mother wipes me dry.

Five days ago I was changing babies' diapers in the NICU.

"It's time we get you up," a physical therapist says, rolling a wheelchair up to my bed at Cedars. "What do you think?"

Yes. Today is the day.

As the therapist elevates the head of the bed, my vertebrae feel stuck, as if they are superglued together. "There's something wrong with my back."

"You're just stiff," she assures me. "You'll be okay."

"I don't know about this," I say. If forced to stretch, I worry my vertebrae will snap and I'll be paralyzed.

"It's only for an hour," she says. "Come on. I'll be right here to help."

As a nurse, I understand the routine followed by healthcare workers. They haul you out of bed as soon as possible, so your muscles don't wither and your lungs don't fill up with fluid and mucus from lying down for too long.

"Okay," I say. "Here I go." I lean forward, the muscles around my spine tugging, tightening, slowly loosening.

"I'm going to swing your legs over the bed now," the therapist says.

As my legs hang over the edge of the mattress, silver circles spin before my eyes, like flipping coins. "I'm dizzy."

"I'm not surprised. You've been in bed for six days. Sit here for a minute." The therapist holds both my arms in her warm hands. "How about if we have you sit up in bed for a while, then try again a little later?"

"No, the dizziness isn't that bad. I'm just a little light-headed." There's a lot of my life I have to get back to: work, running, music. From across the room my fiddle case draws my attention, its solid presence like a faithful partner. I love its pear-shaped body, its slender neck, and curlicue F holes. I also get off on the scent of the varnished wood and the feel of the smooth chinrest against my chin. But the real reason I chose the fiddle: it has no frets, which makes it a difficult instrument to play. If I can master the fiddle, that means I am talented, capable, smart.

I first learned playing the fiddle at age ten. I practiced "Twinkle, Twinkle Little Star" and "Mary Had a Little Lamb" every evening, usually in my bedroom, sparing my family the dreadful sounds of a beginner fiddler. If I missed a note or two, I'd start over, practicing for as long as it took to finish the song without making a mistake. I didn't care that my fingertips throbbed from pressing down on the metal strings for thirty minutes. I'd keep playing.

My father would dutifully listen to me play on the evenings before a recital. Funny how I remember details of these command performances. Me, in my brown corduroy jumper and penny loafers, pretending I was performing for a full house. As I played, my father would fidget in his seat, his fingers near his ears, ready to plug them whenever I bowed a painful note.

After a few minutes, he'd say, "Sounds good," and give me a brief applause while rising to stand, my danger signal that he had had enough. I was afraid of my father, a short-tempered man. To be safe was to do no wrong around him, to be obedient, to never test his patience. When he'd stand up and clap, I'd put on my costume smile and walk back to my bedroom to practice.

By the end of that school year, I lost interest in playing the fiddle, and returned the rented instrument to the music department.

It took me twenty-five years to pick up the fiddle again. Mostly, I was desperate to find an escape from the man I had been living with for the past five years. He was a screamer who scared the hairs on my big toe. In any tense discussion, I did not dare fight back with my voice. He would yell at me for not cutting an onion the "right" way, and once even raised a butcher knife at me.

If we couldn't get along, maybe the fiddle and I could. At least it wouldn't scream back at me, even if the out-of-tune notes did sound like a pissed-off hawk. That could be fixed, though, with a shift of a finger here, another shift there. The strings would bend with my fingers; my fingers would bend with the strings.

I wanted to learn classical, but the only recommended teacher in the area taught Irish music. I walked into my first lesson intent on learning a jig. At thirty-five, maybe it was late to be relearning how to play the fiddle, but I welcomed the new challenge. Although it scared the shit out of me, I also wanted to play at pubs and in music sessions. But during my first lesson, I discovered I was a long way from playing anything.

My instructor spent much of the hour teaching me how to hold the fiddle. "If you don't hold it correctly, you won't play correctly." All I needed to hear was "correctly," an adverb I had so often spoken, and which had been repeatedly spoken to me, even before I learned to talk.

I followed her instructions: "Rest the fiddle on your left shoulder. No. No. Like this. That's it. OK, lower your chin until it sits on the chinrest. Sit up a little straighter like me. OK, hold the fingerboard between your thumb and forefinger. OK, you're getting it."

It was a new relationship, and it would be a while before I felt as if the fiddle and I belonged together. For every new tune my instructor taught me, such as my first Irish polka, she recorded herself playing it, first at full tempo, then at a slower pace. At home, I listened to her recordings over and over, etching the melody's tracks in my brain. I was learning a new language, as if I were dating an Italian guy—sexy, and with a mysterious accent.

At home, I practiced every day, with no one else around to torture. The sounds of an aggravated hawk continued for a while, but my fiddle instructor promised it would get better.

"Keep playing, every day, and you'll train your ear."

Sometimes I'd stamp my clogs against the hardwood living room floor, oblivious to the tenant below, the rhythm sweeping through my feet, into my legs, torso, and arms.

—

I come out of my daydream and look at my pitiful legs hanging over the bed.

"I want you to get up," the physical therapist says. "But if you're too dizzy ..."

"No. I'm not. Please, let's do this."

With the hospital gown hanging off my wasted shoulders, I teeter at the edge of the bed for several seconds, the room swaying, the floor shifting. I breathe in and out, breathing my topsy-turvy world back into focus. As I hold my eyes on the fiddle in the corner, we count together: "One, two, three, up." She carries most of the load, hoists and pivots me ninety degrees, then gently eases me into the wheelchair.

"Just for an hour," she reminds me. "I'll be back."

I lean against the back of the wheelchair, wincing as each vertebra pulls and stretches. I try to let my whole body relax, but my vertebrae pull and stretch even more. I stare steadily at the bold numbers on the manhole-sized clock. The second hand rotates at sloth speed around its mechanical face. *The goal: large hand on the twelve, small hand on the one. One hour. Sixty minutes. Too many seconds to count.*

After what feels like two hours, with the clock showing the large hand on the twelve, I press the call bell.

Chapter 8

I begin to keep track of my independent firsts. Getting in and out of bed: *Do reverse plank. Use arms to lift up from mattress. Pivot forty-five degrees so spine faces seat of wheelchair. Shimmy backwards until butt lands in seat. Wheel a few inches back and swing legs down off bed.*

I accomplish each one of those moves after the physical therapist instructs me how to execute transfers. Four days have passed since I've pressed the call bell.

"Shit," I murmur to the therapist. "Sorry."

I'm a perpetual apologizer, sometimes to the point of annoying others. I even apologize to inanimate objects. "Sorry," I say after knocking over a saltshaker.

"I didn't mean to do that," I say to the physical therapist. I'm sorry for pressing my feet against the footrests of the wheelchair as I demonstrated transferring myself back into bed. For my pelvis to fully heal without the aid of screws or pins, the surgeons cautioned me to be careful of burdening it with my body weight. Which means no pushing with my feet. But training your feet to be still is like training yourself not to scratch an itch.

Everything that I once took for granted as simple, like getting dressed, was now difficult.

The therapist lays out a t-shirt and pair of shorts at the end of the bed. "I'll be back soon to help you put these on," she says, wagging a finger at me.

With the clothes right there, only inches away from me, I can't resist. After she leaves, I reach forward in the bed, and pull the t-shirt toward me. *Closer, closer. Got it.* I strip off the hospital gown, slip on the shirt.

Clogs clamor in the hallway. I fall back against the pillow, wait another minute, listening for more clogs. Ten minutes pass. Twenty. I snatch the shorts. The backs of my legs start sweating. Raising my right leg, I slide one pant leg over it. As I raise my casted leg with the broken foot, I tilt to the side, nearly toppling off the bed. I grip the sheets with one hand and pull the other pant leg over the cast.

I jiggle my hips side to side, pull the shorts all the way up to my belly button. The elastic waist presses against the staples holding me together—a mark of my ruptured spleen. I blow on the skin, fan my hand over the area.

The skin around the staples itches. This itch no one can stop me from attending to. I pick at the edges of each staple, poke them, rub them. Anything to stop the itch. I want to dig my nails into my skin, scratch deep down, into the dermal layer. *This is why dogs wear cones.*

The clogs grow closer, louder. I keep picking, poking, rubbing. The clogs squeak to a stop at the doorway. My eyes lock on hers.

"You got yourself dressed," the therapist says. She claps. "Good for you."

Oh, how much I need to hear that complimentary phrase. "Good for you" equals "Good girl... you're so helpful... so well-behaved." And voila, I forget about the itch, at least for the moment.

When I wake one morning to pain swelling behind my naval, it feels as if I'm about to shit a barbell. It takes all I have in me to breathe and I can't transfer myself out of bed to the commode nearby. It's 6:30 in the morning, a half-hour before change of shift at LA General. Eight, maybe nine, days have passed since I've had a bowel movement. My stomach is as round as a cantaloupe.

I press the call button, hoping a nurse or an aide, anyone—a custodian, a visitor of another patient—will show up soon to retrieve the bedpan in the bathroom. A male nurse arrives. *Yikes.* I can't help but notice his sea-green eyes and dimpled smile. My face blooms red; I can feel the heat. I hope he believes it's from the pain and not utter humiliation. *He's a nurse. He does this all the time, every day, probably in his sleep.*

"Sorry to bother you," I say, "but I need to go, really go."

He pulls on a pair of rubber gloves. *Remember, Melissa. Your ass is not the only one he's seen.*

I use my arms for leverage to roll myself to the side. My body feels as if it's filled with tar. The good-looking nurse slides the bedpan against my butt cheek and I flop back onto the pan like a slab of bologna.

"Take your time," he says. "I'll be right back."

In a semi-reclined position, I clench the side rails and push. My gut boils. I'm terrified all twenty-four staples lining my belly will loosen and my insides will spill out. Dehiscence: the splitting open of a surgical wound. I pant and purse-lip breathe, like I learned to do in nursing school during my labor and delivery rotation.

I start perspiring and my hands keep slipping off the side rail each time I push and grunt. Finally, my bowels pop and empty, then empty some more.

Fifteen minutes, maybe longer, pass before my bowels stop contracting. Now sitting in a mound of moist shit, I remember what my mother said moments before she left for the airport a day ago.

"Maybe I shouldn't leave."

"No, you've done enough," I insisted.

She kissed me on the forehead, and walked toward the door, her head down, then turned back. "Are you sure?"

"I'm OK," I said. "Really."

But now, sitting in my own shit, I wish my mother were here to wipe me, though it would probably be less humiliating to have a perfect stranger clean up my mess, someone who would forget my name and face as soon as I left the hospital and he was called to wipe someone else's ass. But not a perfect handsome male stranger. No fucking way.

I reach for the full box of tissues on the bedside table. "Two-Ply" on the label is misleading; more like half-ply. I use all forty tissues. I then roll onto my side, and with one hand carefully slide the bedpan out from underneath me. I reach over the side of the bed, set the pan on the floor, swipe a towel from the bedside table, and toss it over the mound. Moments later, the hot-looking nurse returns.

—

Taking my first shower two weeks after the accident ranks pretty damn close to having an orgasm. With my casted leg wrapped in plastic, I let the warm water pour onto my head, stream down my neck, my shoulders, my back, massage me between my legs. I lather my hair with a handful of shampoo, dig my fingernails into my scalp, scratch deep, deeper. With the soap, I rub my arms and legs, my breasts and belly, scrub between my fingers and toes. I look closely at my body, touch the healing wound on my thigh, the puncture to my calf, run my hands along the yellowing bruises, studying them for texture and depth.

I feel buoyant, held up by a wide blue lake. I open my mouth up to the water showering down on me. It tastes sweet, like well water. I run my tongue over my gums, mmming and aahing. I stay in the shower for a long time, indifferent to my shriveled fingers and toe pads. I curl my toes up tightly, and hold onto the water.

Chapter 9

A physical therapist pushes a brand-new wheelchair into my hospital room at Cedars-Sinai Medical Center, where I will spend the next eight days in rehab.

"This one should be much more comfortable than the hospital wheelchairs you've been using," she says.

I reach out to touch the vinyl-coated seat. It off-gasses with the odor of plastic. I then run my hand along the steel armrests. They're cold, as if they have been stored in an unheated warehouse for a long time. And the tires are as narrow as a hula hoop. I wonder if they'll pop under the constant weight of me.

"Do you want to go for a spin in it?" the therapist asks, as if she were encouraging me to test drive a new car. The mental image of driving hits me head on, bulldozes me backward in the bed. Will I ever be able to trust other drivers again, no matter their age? Will I be able to trust myself as a driver?

"I guess I should try it," I say.

Using a new maneuver I recently learned to transfer in and out of the hospital chair, I pivot myself around on the bed, reach with one hand for the far arm of the wheelchair, then grab the other arm, and drop like a sack of mud into the seat.

"How is it?" the therapist asks.

I wiggle this way and that way, the seat sticking to me, then unsticking from me, as if someone is rolling an adhesive lint remover across my naked butt. The seat is as thin as a plastic platter, the armrests restricting, the backrest hard. I'll have to modify the chair somehow to my liking. What other choice do I have, other than waiting out the three months in bed, the amount of time the surgeons said it would take for my pelvis to heal? I had to think of the chair as my Get-Out-of-Jail-Free card.

As I readjust my casted foot and leg so that they fit the footplates, I think about the last time I went for a run: seventeen days ago. How easy it was for me then to lace up my sneakers, dash down the stairs of my apartment in Montpelier and out the door in the direction of the murmuring Winooski River, the soft breeze brushing my face, the scent of freshly mowed hay as I ran along the sun-warmed bike path. I was unstoppable.

Now, from my vantage point in the wheelchair, that day seems like an age ago, an ultra-marathon away. I haven't worn sneakers, or any kind of shoes, in seventeen days. Shoes are of little value while in a wheelchair. The footplates of the chair are now my shoes. I reposition my feet again, the aluminum shocking the sole of my uncasted foot like tinfoil on a tooth.

I imagine the day when I'll be walking again, like I imagined riding a real bike when I was a child, dreaming the training wheels away. Pink-and-yellow tassels tied to the handlebars flap up and down as if they are waving at me. My legs are nimble, strong, quick. Birds whistle and trill from treetops. Some swoop down from branches to fly along with me, their wings beating in rhythm, it seems, with the circling of my legs. I arch my neck back, glimpsing a fine gathering of clouds ribboning a blue sky.

When a physical therapist suggests I practice wheeling my chair across an intersection outside of Cedars, I'm not sure I can trust my arms to rotate the tires as fast as my feet and legs once rotated the pedals of my bicycle. I wait for a wink, or a smirk, any kind of facial gesture indicating she is not serious.

"Let's go," she says.

Fear punches me in the gut. I lose my breath for a moment. *She's out of her blasted mind.* But I can't refuse. Nurses don't say no—"Sure, I'll work a double shift." Besides, I need to know I can cross the intersection. I need to know I can get to the other side.

From waist level in a wheelchair, everything appears much bigger: motor vehicles, tires, headlights. I used to feel safe walking across a street. I trusted my feet to move fast when the walk signal flashed with only two seconds left before the light turned green. But, now, when I see the four-way intersection congested with cars, I say, "You want me to wheel across *this* street?"

"I'll be right beside you," she says, "the entire way."

"What if the cars don't stop?"

"The cars will stop, I promise."

Like a prayer, I whisper, "Promise, promise, promise."

With the therapist at my side, we wait at the edge of the crosswalk for the traffic light to turn red and the walk signal to flash. Wearing bicycle gloves to protect my palms, I seize each wheel, ready to propel across the zebra-striped lines. The line of traffic creeps to a stop, engines idling. Their grilles are like tiger teeth within inches of us. Front windshields reflect the blistering sun. Exhaust fumes poison the air. Finally, the walk signal flashes.

"Ready," the therapist says. "Go."

I turn my head right, then left, wheel across the street, summoning all my energy to cycle my arms as fast as they can move. The veins in my forearms bulge. Sweat drips down my neck. I continue rolling ahead, my eyes trained toward my destination—the level sidewalk—not once allowing myself to be diverted by headlights, their chrome grilles radiating tiger-breath heat. Pure adrenaline pushes me along. I can't feel my arms or hands.

My strength wanes as I bang into the curb on the other side of the crosswalk. My body whips forward then backward.

"I can't get over it." My voice rises in panic.

The therapist grabs the handlebars of the chair, popping a wheelie over the curb. "It's okay. When you're back in Vermont, others will help you. Didn't you say you'd be living with friends for a while?"

I want to ask her why she pushed me into such a frightening place, a place where I felt so out of control. But I don't.

Instead, I say, "Yes, you're right."

Yes, I will be living with friends. Yes, others will help me. But traffic lights, walk signals—and drivers—can't be trusted. I'm not even sure I can trust the wheelchair. The world is dangerous. At any given moment, anything could be smashed apart.

Chapter 10

It would take me years to begin to trust myself and the world enough to cross an intersection without fear of being run down. It would take years before I could see an older driver behind the wheel of a car and not shudder and wonder if the driver was another Russell Weller.

Our deepest fears can rule our lives. They can make us hide and deny, like a child burying oneself beneath a pile of pillows, hoping the boogeyman won't find her. But sometimes we choose to study our fear, to examine its causes and learn how to protect ourselves and others from getting hurt.

Eventually, I'd become a student of the little-understood phenomenon known as "pedal error," an oddly sanitized and trivializing label for something that begins with a moment of confusion yet ends with blood on concrete. The more I learned, the more I understood that what had happened to me had happened to so many others, and would continue happening, because little was being done to tackle the root causes or prevent its recurrence.

In April 1992, a class field trip turned into a horror show at Chicago's O'Hare International Airport. An eighty-seven-year-old, driving a Delta 88 Oldsmobile, jumped a curb at the terminal entrance, smashing into a group of third graders, the impact scattering bodies and hurling people onto the hood. The car stopped when it slammed into a pole, the tires still spinning. The carnage—a dead nine-year-old, dozens of others injured, some critically.

The driver, Martin Horvath, told police officers the accelerator of his car stuck. But investigators found nothing wrong with the car. Horvath had stepped on the gas pedal instead of the brake. "This is just an extremely unfortunate accident," a traffic investigator said, only hours later.

In August 2012, a one-hundred-year-old driver backed his Cadillac into a group of students leaving a Los Angeles elementary school, injuring eleven children and three adults. The driver told reporters that the brakes had failed.

In April 2019, a man in his eighties confused the gas pedal for the brake and struck pedestrians at a congested intersection in Tokyo, killing a mother and her two-year-old daughter.

In April 2025, a ninety-three-year-old man in Pike, Ohio, ran a stop sign. The driver survived her injuries, but the passenger, a ninety-five-year-old woman, did not.

People are aging and living longer. Which means they are driving longer. Which means it will keep happening—the "extremely unfortunate" pedal error.

Chapter 11

Her name is Tina. Like a newly-remembered dream, her sudden presence in my hospital room at Cedars triggered a whirl of fuzzy images: people wearing white coats or blue scrubs rushing past me, stethoscopes swaying around necks, mechanical voices talking from the ceiling. I did not remember it at the time, but Tina had knelt by my side as I lay on the hot asphalt at the Farmers' Market. She was the woman with the berry-red lips in that morphine dream the day of the accident.

She walks toward me, leans down, and hugs me snugly, the way you would hug a long-time friend. The scent of a flower garden surrounds me. "Melissa, you look great."

I give her a weak smile, accepting her kind lie. I feel like I must look like a bag of gashes and bruises, all purple and mustard-colored.

"I mean, that day I saw you at the hospital," Tina says," you were so pale and weak."

"That's right, you were staring down at me." I search my mind and try to locate exactly where in the hospital I saw Tina. *The emergency room?* More memories collide. The edges of Tina's long brown hair brushing my shoulder. Flickering lights. A hard, cold stretcher. Sterile, frigid odors.

"I had no idea which hospital the rescue workers were taking you to," Tina says. "I called all the emergency rooms in the area. When I finally found you at the hospital, you were lying on a stretcher in a hallway. At the accident scene, you kept repeating the names of family members, where they lived, and their phone numbers. 'My dad lives in Florida, my mother lives in Massachusetts, my dad lives in Florida, my mother lives in Massachusetts.'"

Tina might as well be talking about someone else. It's as if I was not present at the scene of the accident.

"I don't remember any of that," I say.

"Let me start at the beginning," Tina says. "For some reason, I decided to walk a different route to the Farmers' Market for lunch. As I moved to step off the curb onto Arizona, a car sped by me. My hair went flying from the wind of the car." She flips her hair up high to demonstrate.

My hands shoot up over my gaping mouth. I can't bring myself to say it out loud: *What if she was hit?*

"Oh my God, Tina, how close were you to the market?"

She sits down on the bed, reaches for her purse on the floor, and combs through it for a piece of paper and a pen.

From the wheelchair, I watch her sketch the accident scene. She scribbles out a rough map, and with a red-polished fingernail, shows me an X. "Right about here," she says, and drags her nail, showing the direction the driver came from.

"I ran after the car. There were people and vendor stands down everywhere. She slides her finger along the map. "You were lying *right here*, in front of a collapsed fruit stand."

Tina points at a spot on the floor beside the wheelchair, explaining that a person lay next to me on the sidewalk covered in blood, screaming. Then she points at my feet as she describes how another person lay with her legs mangled and twisted in the wrong direction. I close my eyes, but cannot retreat from the gruesome details. I see blood, puddles of blood.

I wonder about my own blood. *How much was left on the pavement? Where did it go? Did it swirl down a sewer drain? Or maybe my blood fed into the puddles. What happened to those two people lying next to me? Did they die?* Tina quiets, sensing I need to process this mind-bending horror.

I open my eyes and look down at my hands, at the bruise circling my wrist. It was probably caused by the watch I wore that day. The rescue workers had saved it, sealed it in a Ziploc bag, along with some dried blood. *The two victims who lay so close to me: Is some of their blood in that bag? What are their names? What do they look like?*

What about the driver? Where was he? I envision a hunched-back man with a wrinkled face and cataract eyes. I don't know his name. I haven't yet heard his name spoken in the news: George Russell Weller. Russell Weller. Weller. I've been avoiding watching television. Listening to Tina share the details is one thing, but to risk seeing the grim images of the accident scene will make the horror too real.

I surface from my reverie. Tina is staring at me. "Why did you choose me?" I ask. After long, silent seconds pass, she says, "You sent energy out to me—a message."

I study her face for meaning. *What kind of energy? What message?*

"If you weren't there, I don't know what would've happened," I say.

"Melissa, you saved yourself." Tina sees my puzzled expression. "You didn't allow yourself to die. I might have run past you, but you reached up from the pavement for the cuff of my blouse. You cried out, 'Please, don't let me die.'"

I force my chest and belly to expand, filling all of me with new air.

"I found your nursing I.D. in the pocket of your shorts," Tina says, feeling for her own pockets. "I wasn't surprised to learn that you're a nurse because you kept repeating the name of the hospital where you work, and the names of friends, people to contact, as though you knew what information was important to tell me." I clamp my eyes shut, now wanting to remember, wanting to hear the voice inside of the other me—the one sprawled on the pavement.

"You kept trying to sit up," she says. "You lifted up your shirt to take it off. You said, 'My back is burning.'"

"I kept telling you, 'Don't take off your shirt, help is on the way.' I panicked. I screamed at the people standing by the windows of the building across the street to bring me water. Then you started saying your back hurt. I put my hand under it. It was swollen. I looked and saw all the bruises. You started to turn gray. I grabbed the arm of a firefighter as he passed me and yelled, 'She's not okay.' He knelt down and I showed him your back."

I shift in the wheelchair, trying to relieve the pricking sensation shooting down my spine.

"You had a green tag on your toe," Tina continues. "For stable. The firefighter ripped it off and tagged you with a red one, for urgent."

I suddenly understand that without Tina I would have died, right there, with a green tag on my toe.

"How many others do you think were injured?" I ask.

"I think sixty or seventy, maybe more. It was carnage. The City of Santa Monica held a memorial service for the ten who died."

I drop my head into my clammy hands. *Ten.* I had heard that ten died.

"Hundreds of people showed up for the service," Tina says. "There was a shrine with flowers, and a lit candle for each of the ten victims. People left cards, letters, and prayers. They tacked them onto a huge board."

"I wish I could've been there."

"Melissa, no one expected you to be at the service," Tina says, her voice lulling. "You needed to heal. You still do."

Chapter 12

A few days after Tina's visit, she returns with her eleven-year-old son, Brett. He has a present for me: a teddy bear. After they leave, I brush my face against his silky, soft body, the taffeta bow tickling my cheek. I cuddle into his neck, trying to hide from the mangled legs, the toe tags. The Buick. The bear smells familiar, like woods, leaves, Vermont. I bury my nose deeper into his plush neck.

—

Healing takes time; at least, that's what we're told. Our broken bones will one day mend, our bruises will fade, and our scars will become a tender reminder of a misfortune recorded in the visible history of our bodies—a landmark commemorating a trauma we endured and overcame. The body remembers, yet tethers us to the now. But the mind is a compulsive time traveler, flitting from the present to the future and venturing unbidden into the past. Years later, long after recovering from my physical injuries, I remain susceptible to trauma-inducing, real-world intrusions that come mostly in the form of news reports of innocent people mowed down by out-of-control drivers. And I find myself reliving the past.

It's the summer of 2016, when images of a vehicle-ramming attack flash across the television screen. I don't want to watch the mayhem unfolding, but I can't stop myself. A man had rented a cargo truck and barreled along a seafront promenade, into a crowd celebrating Bastille Day in Nice. He killed eighty-six people. Ten of the dead are children. I have trouble focusing on the details of the story, but I get the gist of it: a Tunisian man had "answered the calls" of ISIS (Islamic State of Iraq and Syria) urging would-be terrorists to target citizens of nations working to combat terrorism. The final toll of the injured—a catastrophic 458.

The ground gives way beneath me, and with a nauseating lurch of my stomach, I think I might vomit. My email's inbox fills up with one "I'm-thinking-of-you" message after another, with "I hope you're okay…I hope you're well." No, I am not okay. I have no idea if I'll ever be okay again.

What I did not know after the Farmers' Market crash—what I could not know—was that the coming decades would be marred by a global vehicle-ramming epidemic. Vehicle-ramming incidents, also known as vehicle as a weapon or VAW attack, have become a disturbing worldwide trend. From Charlottesville to New York City and Ohio State University. From Ontario to London and Berlin. If you type in "vehicle-ramming" you'll find a Wikipedia entry listing one attack after the next.

Of all the vehicle-ramming attacks occurring around that time, the Nice incident delivered the hardest blow to my sense of peace. It happened on July 14, two days before the thirteenth anniversary of the Santa Monica Farmers' Market crash. As with each anniversary during those thirteen years, for weeks I prepared myself. Each morning, I looked at the flip calendar hanging on my refrigerator, and marked the countdown in my head: *June 30, July 1, July 5, July 12.*

The 14th.

At 11 p.m. local time, the driver turned terrorist began his death hunt.

2 p.m. in Santa Monica.

Thirteen minutes after Russell Weller had pressed down on the gas pedal. No, he did not intend to kill or harm people, but the moment he barreled past the Do Not Enter sign, his car became a weapon. All it took was twenty seconds. Ten dead. In a matter of seconds, the Santa Monica Farmers' Market went from an idyllic place to one that resembled a terrorist car-bombing attack.

No, I was not okay.

I was terrified of what would come next: if the next vehicle-ramming attack would happen here in Vermont. If the next news headline would read, "Ten Killed in Burlington." What the next knock on my door, or phone call I'd receive would be. I still can't bring myself to retell the kind of terror scenarios my head came up with that day.

In an email sent to me the day after the Nice incident, a friend writes, "I've been thinking of you, because, though this seems deliberately done, and the Farmers' Market was an accident, they have a similar style and tragedy."

Too similar. Alarmingly similar. They are still similar.

Motorized vehicles are everywhere. And how easy it is, despite intention, age, or experience of the driver, for a vehicle to become a lethal weapon—a means of inflicting mass casualties. At any given moment, a car, an SUV, or an eighteen-wheeler could bear down on any one of us.

Every muscle in my body contracts when I think about the mounting death toll resulting from each successive incident involving vehicle-ramming attacks and mass-casualty accidents in which a driver mows down pedestrians. "The city is safe," the Toronto police chief said in response to the deadliest rampage involving a vehicle in Canada. In April 2018, ten people were killed, mostly women, and another sixteen injured, when a troubled loner deliberately drove a white rental Ryder van along Toronto's main artery during a busy lunch hour. The driver—Alek Minassian—intentionally struck one pedestrian after the other, tossing people into the street, crushing others in crosswalks, pinning a woman beneath the van. Nearly one-and-a-half miles later, his killing spree came to a stop.

Once again, the Toronto attack bore an eerie resemblance to what had happened in Santa Monica in terms of the carnage. But not in terms of the drivers. I wanted to try to understand what motivated a man like Minassian—a twenty-year-old college student who had been bullied as a kid for his Asperger's, and later discharged from the Canadian Armed Forces sixteen days after being recruited. His rancor eventually led him to the toxic, social media realm of so-called "incels" (short for involuntary celibates), a radical hate group made up of frustrated and misogynistic young men who blame women, especially young attractive ones, for their feelings of isolation and sexual inadequacy.

How does such pure madness, a gross act of outrage, leave those who were enjoying an outdoor lunch under the sun-sweetened skies of Toronto feeling at all safe? Does the bystander who rushed to help a pedestrian struck while crossing the street feel safe? And what about the injured, or the families of the dead?

Learning of the Toronto attack, I knew all too well they would never feel safe again. Maybe they, too, still mistrust walk signals, traffic lights, all cars, all drivers. I imagine their feet coming to a cold stop at the edge of a curb, their feet refusing to move into the crosswalk each time they see a white Ryder van waiting for a traffic light to turn green. Just as my feet freeze solid to the innermost edge of the sidewalk whenever I see a Buick Le Sabre idling at a stop light.

The memorial service for all of those who died in Santa Monica was held on July 23, one week after the accident. Other, smaller services were held. Also, on July 23, family and friends gathered for a memorial for Lynne, a Native American advocate and environmental activist whose favorite flowers were hydrangeas, favorite drink Champagne, and favorite music 1960s roots rock. She was remembered for her first-and-foremost priority: her daughter,

Jennifer, and husband, Robby Weaver, son of actor Dennis Weaver. She had been at the market to purchase fresh ingredients for Robby, the accomplished cook in the family, when the Buick took her.

On July 21, Diana and Kevin were remembered: Diana, a classical pianist, singer, and designer; Kevin, a filmmaker and literary wizard. Colleagues of Diana's at the Skirball Cultural Center, where she worked part-time welcoming visitors, spoke of her as "warm, kind, funny." Her graceful presence and professional experience made her one of those rare people who make the perfect fit for a culture-focused non-profit. A long-time friend of Kevin's remembered the slim, bespectacled man for his love of discussing books, art, and politics. And for having "a thousand ideas." One of those ideas: "The Rogue Shoes." The silent film, a comedy based on Hans Christian Andersen's tale, "The Red Shoes," features a ballerina whose life is transformed when her wish to dance before an audience comes true. Kevin and Diana's wish was to someday see the comedy on the big screen. But the Buick came after them first, and Kevin's interview with a major film studio never happened. That interview had been scheduled for the following day.

Brandon and his grandmother, Molok, who had been wheeling him across Arizona Avenue in search of produce for the upcoming Jewish Sabbath, were memorialized on July 20. Some 750 people attended their funeral at Eden Memorial Park cemetery in Mission Hills. Molok and Brandon are buried in the park, side-by-side.

The day before the city's service, investigators released the name of one of the deceased victims previously withheld: Theresa Breglia. A slender fifty-year-old woman, she wore a cotton pouch wrapped around her waist, containing only bus tokens and a New York driver's license. For five days, no one, neither family nor friends, came looking for her. No one claimed her body. Investigators made phone calls to both the Bronx, New York, address noted on her license and to the Moreno Valley one on record. They came up empty-handed. Police visited the Bronx address, but there was no answer. Newspapers and television stations made her face public. After scrolling through a database of credit reports and property records, investigators eventually located her sister in New York and gave her the shocking news. Theresa had struggled for years with mental illness, and had lived with her sister in the Bronx until a month before the accident, when she relocated to the LA area with the hope of reuniting with her ex-husband. That hope was crushed by a Buick on a hot day on Arizona Avenue.

Chapter 13

Wearing a sports coat, necktie, and a crisply ironed collar, Mr. Archer, the attorney my father contacted, walks up to my bedside at Cedars. He sets his briefcase down on the floor, and as he shakes my hand, smiling, the earthy scent of his leather case slows my galloping heart to a canter. It further slows, settling into a trot, when he pulls a chair close to my bed and asks how I am feeling. He even apologizes when he has done nothing wrong. "I'm so sorry this happened to you." But when he says he wants to ask me questions about the accident, I'm afraid my heart will leap from my chest. To answer those questions is to relive the crash.

Like an attentive teacher, he articulates every word. "What do you remember? What kind of injuries did you sustain? How long have you been a nurse? What kind of activities did you enjoy before the accident?" As I answer him as best as I can, his eyes shift from my face to his notepad, his pencil tip hurrying across the page. During the occasional pause when Mr. Archer studies his notes and rubs his graying beard, I wonder what he is thinking. What exactly is he writing? I feel I am not being helpful, since I have no memory of the Buick heading toward me, of being slammed to the ground, my head meeting the pavement, my ribs cracking, my pelvis shattering. No memory of the blood and sirens and screams.

Mr. Archer looks up from his pad. "I know, this must be hard for you." He takes a breath, then says he will file a claim against the City of Santa Monica and the other entities responsible for the running and safety of the Farmers' Market. At the time of the accident, only plastic orange-and-white striped barriers blocked traffic from three side streets, including Second, onto Arizona Avenue.

"Russell Weller won't be named in the civil suit," Mr. Archer says. "He'll likely face criminal charges. Possibly murder, but most likely manslaughter."

I sit upright in the bed, my leg cast throwing me off balance. I latch onto the pillow next to me for support. *A murderer? But didn't someone—Tina?—say Russell Weller believed he was stepping on the brake? That doesn't make him a murderer. Who is this man?*

"Are you okay?" Mr. Archer asks.

"Yeah," I lie, and collapse back onto the mattress.

"This will be a lengthy case," he says, and tucks his notepad into his briefcase. Zips it shut. Snaps together the copper buttons. "Why don't you think about things. Give me a call when you're settled back in Vermont."

Mr. Archer stands up and shakes my hand. As he picks up his briefcase, another scent of leather drifts toward me. He walks away, and the scent dissipates. I want to be inside that briefcase, with the zipper shut and the buttons clasped. I want to be tucked inside a place where there's an insular lining, away from everything real, like deciding whether I have permission to be angry, or if the correct thing is to forgive someone who merely made a mistake and didn't intentionally mean to hurt me. Inside that briefcase, I'd never have to decide these things. I'd never have to worry whether it's okay to step between the white lines to cross the street.

After Mr. Archer's visit, a good friend calls me. I tell him about Mr. Archer, that I'm not sure I want to be part of a lawsuit. "The man didn't drive through the Farmers' Market on purpose," I say. "Mr. Archer said he confused the gas pedal for the brake."

"That's why people have auto insurance," my friend reminds me. "It's okay for you to sue this guy."

But the word "lawsuit" sounds dirty, like one of the seven deadly sins: greed. It reminds me of one of those slick-haired, seedy characters you see in the movies.

With his voice growing louder as he speaks each word, my friend says "Melissa, you'll never be the same again." His candid tone cuts through the illusionary world in which I have been hiding. No one else has spoken such chilling words to me.

Yet, I want to know more about Russell Weller. I do not believe he is a murderer. I do not want to believe he is a murderer, because that would mean he wanted to kill us. I want to believe Russell Weller is an old guy who made a terrible mistake. But for the first time since the accident, the new truth is, I am angry. I don't know what to do with my anger, though, where to place it. As I lie in bed, I think of how I was never allowed to show my anger growing up, and now I'm not sure if it's okay to feel this way. Anger doesn't fit me, like clothes that are too small. My skin feels tight, as if it has shrunk. It's a claustrophobic feeling. I want to kick the anger out of me, as though I am defending myself against an assailant. I'm afraid it won't stop, like a prolonged violent seizure. I won't be able to hide my blue-flamed rage from others. Hiding my anger keeps me safe.

I don't even know with whom I should be angry. My friend? It's bullshit that I'll never be the same again. The Farmers' Market officials for failing to ensure pedestrian safety? Or Russell Weller for harming us? I don't believe he's a murderer. But I begin to wonder why he had been driving at all. Had someone told him he should not be driving?

Blood samples taken from Russell Weller at the hospital revealed no traces of alcohol or illicit or prescription drugs. A week later, state officials revoked his driver's license for "lack of knowledge and skill." His medical history noted he had bilateral hip replacements in 1993, but that his hips were "stable." He had no history of neurological issues such as seizures or cognitive difficulties.

Though he had no moving violations, he had been in three previous accidents. While backing down a driveway in 1993, he collided with a retaining wall. In 1998, while attempting to park, he hit another parked car multiple times with his front bumper. A year later, one side of his car was struck by another car backing out of a parking lot. Then on that tragic day, July 16, 2003, Russell Weller stopped to mail a letter at a curbside mailbox on Fifth Street in Santa Monica. After pulling away from the curb, he turned right onto Arizona Avenue and rear-ended a Mercedes-Benz that had stopped at Fourth Street to let pedestrians cross. He swerved around the car, apparently unaware he had hit it, picking up speed as he confused the gas pedal for the brake, and plunged through the market—at sixty miles an hour.

Chapter 14

The visible remains of the accident on my body—the hurricane-shaped tear on my hand, the crescent moon gash on my thigh, and the half-dollar puncture to my calf—bring back the various memories of the scars imprinted on the bodies and minds of the burned children I cared for as a nurse at Shriners Hospitals for Children in Boston years ago. Images, smells, and sounds swirl: cauterized tissue souring the air, a child's leathered fingers feeling for my latex-gloved hands, ventilators blowing into smoke-filled lungs. *Pshhh hooo, pshhh, hooo.*

The three-year-old boy whose cousin had doused him in gasoline then lit him on fire is as present as my own heartbeat. For weeks, a battery of medical equipment—intravenous pumps, ventilator, arterial blood pressure line, cardiac and oxygen monitor—kept him alive. So did the decisions made by the nurses and doctors: when to tweak a ventilator button, titrate the morphine drip, or adjust the oxygen level.

During each of my twelve-hour shifts, as I changed his full-body dressings, slowly unraveling the yellowish-green stained gauze, I'd talk to him. "It'll be over soon. You'll be okay. I promise, sweetie." I remember how making that promise helped me now. I, too, need it to be over soon.

His eyes were one of the few places on his body not burned. They appeared black next to all the white gauze cocooned around his tiny head. Sometimes his eyes would twitch side to side, as if he were trying to speak through them, signaling to me he wanted, needed, something. To distract him from his fear and confusion, I'd roll the television close to him and slip a video into the DVD player so he could watch Barney giggle, dance, and sing. Other times, I'd slide a CD of lullabies into the boom box on the shelf above his bed. I'd hum along to the music as I wrapped him in fresh white, forming a figure-eight pattern around his arms and legs. Every two hours, I sprinkled warmed-up antibacterial solution over his limbs and chest and back, the white bandages turning a grayish-brown. These dressing changes often took two hours. But each time I finished the task, I felt relieved at the sight of a newly wrapped little boy, now a step closer to being healed. I knew he felt relief when his eyes drifted in their sockets, slowly blinking, his lids halfway closing with the onset of a long, deep sleep, then closing all the way, like window blinds drawn against a maddening glare.

The four-year-old girl from Haiti I cared for in 1993 came to Shriners with a patchwork of scars covering fifty percent of her body. She needed multiple surgeries to release constricted tissue from burns sustained months earlier. Because she was a host of contagious infections, we kept her isolated in her own room. On the day of her admission, I approached her crib, wearing a gown, surgical cap, and face mask, prepared to change her dressings. She erupted with a gurgling scream, and batted at me as if she were swatting a fly.

"Okay, okay," I tried to assure her. But she spoke French, not one word of English. I slid down the bars of the crib; she scooted to one corner, looking away from me. "My name is Melissa." I spoke slowly, as if doing so would help her decipher my English. She eyed me; I reached out for her. She looked away again, now clinging to the bars. I tried once more, this time slipping off my mask so she could see more of me. She smiled, a shy smile. I reached for her doll at the end of the crib, and started wrapping one leg in gauze. The little girl shifted closer toward me. But when I reached out for her arm to show her that I needed to change her dressings, she kicked me, and grabbed her doll, clasping it to her chest.

"Okay, no more for now," I said. "Let's rest." I sat in the rocker by her crib during lunch, watching her chew on chicken wings. Down to the bone. Gnawing into the marrow. When she stopped gnawing, she smiled at me and said, "Monamee (*Mon ami*)." My friend. It's the only French phrase I recall learning during the few months I cared for her. That afternoon, I let her change her doll's dressing first. It worked. She held her arm out and let me change hers. Though it took several hours, I earned her trust.

Who were these children beneath their white pain? Who was I beneath all my black bruises and jagged-edged wounds? In the hospital, I lay in a state of role confusion. No guidebook exists that helps a nurse transition from caregiver to patient. I was smothered in my own white pain and doubt.

Though I'd come to accept my scars taking shape beneath my bandages as a reminder that I had survived, other kinds of scars would matter more. The ones on the inside, the scars no one else could see. My mind conjuring flying bodies when car brakes squeal. Feeling as if my heart has been tasered the moment a fire truck or ambulance siren wails.

Wherever they are, maybe the burn patients I once cared for, those lucky enough to have survived, are at peace with their scars. I pray and hope so.

Chapter 15

The call bells start dinging like a never-ending video game one afternoon on the rehab unit. Instead of trying to nap, I pull out a novel from my dresser drawer next to the bed. I had started reading *The Secret Life of Bees* on my plane trip to California. In the book, the protagonist, Lily, recalls the day she shot her mother. "I accidentally killed her." I can't concentrate; my eye snags on the word "killed." My mind rearranges the letters, changing the word to "liked." "I accidentally liked her." I guess it's possible to accidentally like someone. I read it again; the letters shift back to their original places. "Killed." It has been more than two weeks since the accident, and I am still taking Vicodin for hip and back pain. I think that maybe the drugs are causing me to hallucinate, to see words that aren't there. *Did Russell Weller accidentally like ten people? Would he have liked them if he knew them?*

I slap the book closed and slide it back into the drawer. *Ding, ding, ding.* The call bells won't shut up. I slip on a pair of headphones, turn on the CD player next to the bed, and listen to a meditation, trying to focus like a good Buddha on the tinkling chimes and trickling streams. A supra-soprano chant pierces through me, and the peaceful chimes shift into a random clattering of sounds. I turn off the CD player. Frustrated and cranky, my thoughts cast back to Lily killing her mother, then to the ten people who died at the Farmers' Market. It feels right, like my thoughts belong in this place, with the dead.

During a trauma assessment with a psychiatrist one afternoon, he asks, "Is there anything on your mind you want to tell me?"

Anything on my mind? Any one thing? My mind is a catch-all drawer; I have no idea where to start. Having asked the question, he is silent, looking at me through his geeky professor eyeglasses, his hands folded on his lap. In the quiet, the dinging call bells grow louder, much louder, as if each ding is saying, "Hey, stupid, wake up. Remember, he's a psychiatrist. He knows all about trauma."

"Actually, there's something I've been a little obsessed with." I pause, feeling a little self-absorbed for what I am about to ask.

He leans in. "I'm listening."

What the fuck. Go for it. "Why? How? I mean I can't stop trying to make sense of how or why *I* survived." Embarrassment fills my face with heat. "You must hear that all the time, right?" I'm hoping for a "yes."

He sits back, smiles, as if relieved by the question. Like a magician who pulls a coin out from behind your ear, he conveniently has an answer. "It's survivor's guilt." He holds his steady, certain eyes on mine. "It's normal for survivors of such a tragedy to ask themselves that question."

Shrieks, colliding vendor posts, and fast footsteps all compete with one another in my head. I pull my arms into my chest, rub them, as if I can rub away the noise.

"Over time," he says, "you'll have less feelings of guilt."

How much time? I rub my arms harder, now wanting to rub away the guilt. Believe it or not, though I am a nurse, I have never heard of survivor's guilt, and I'm not sure I believe the psychiatrist's diagnosis. I don't want to believe him. Survivor's guilt sounds like a packaging label for people suffering from something no one can otherwise explain. There must be a reason for my guilt. The psychiatrist's explanation isn't a reason; it doesn't help me deal with it.

Part of my guilt stems from knowing that my fight-or-flight response kicked my primitive emotions into high gear, and I harnessed every bit of my energy to save myself. I came first. No one else mattered. I reached out to Tina and cried, "Please don't let me die," rather than staying still so she could help the other injured pedestrians.

That's why I needed to know what happened to the two people Tina described lying next to me, covered in blood. If I found out that they survived, I'd feel less guilty. If I learned that they had died, I'd feel as if I had contributed to their deaths, thanks to my selfish request for help. Maybe I was supposed to feel guilty, and the psychiatrist didn't want to tell me that. I began to wonder if survivor's guilt was intended for the living as a means to remind us not to forget the dead. As I began to heal, I spent months reading and re-reading the names of the dead in news articles. I memorized all ten. Brandon. Cindy. Gloria. Diana. Lynne. Theresa. Kevin. Leroy. Molok. Movsha.

If survivor's guilt comes with a color, I imagine it being yellow. Yellow forces you to be alert. It calls on you to be aware or to act. A highlighter. Sticky notes. A scorching sun that drives you into the shade. Lemon, the tart bite that reminds you of your canker sore. Flashing traffic lights. Caution tape dividing the living from the dead.

I could not have been alone in that yellow world. There were sixty-two other survivors, and the loved ones of the deceased. Maybe Cindy's mother wished she had tugged her daughter's hand with a little more force, pulling her back off the road, saving her from being dragged away by the Buick's bumper. Maybe Brandon's mother regretted leaving her son and his grandmother on the other side of Arizona Avenue while she crossed the street to get better cell service so she could speak with her sister. And maybe Lynne's husband, Rob, wished he, rather than his wife, had gone to the Farmers' Market to purchase fresh ingredients for the dinner he had planned to make that evening.

It would take years for me to fully understand survivor's guilt—both its tenacity and prevalence—all documented in painful detail in the news stories I read about other survivors of vehicle-ramming attacks. Russell Schulz is only one of many who would later join my yellow world. He climbed out from beneath the rubble of a wine house, surviving the 2016 Christmas market ramming attack in Berlin, Germany. But in the ensuing months, he could not seem to find his way out from the emotional rubble. He'd cry for no apparent reason, and couldn't understand the unfair outcome of what had happened. His friend died in the attack, yet he did not. They were together, at the same time, in the same place, Russell standing only a few inches to the side of his friend. A trauma therapist told him he had survivor's guilt. He urged Russell not to allow empathy to morph into guilt—the two are not one and the same. "Feel empathetic," the therapist said, and encouraged him to write a letter to the friend he lost, then bury it, an act to help him overcome guilt.

Yellow must have surrounded Russell Weller, too. What shade? Muted or electric?

Chapter 16

I'm halfway through my eight days of rehab at Cedars when I cry hard for the first time since the accident nearly three weeks ago. Tears drip into the matzo ball soup before me. I don't think the tears will stop. My parents have already returned to the East Coast. I feel lonely, and a little hurt.

"Are you okay?" a nurse asks, as she walks into my room. She hands me a tissue from a box nearby.

I stare at the crumbling matzo ball. *I'm smashed.*

But really, I was already smashed.

After my parents divorced in 1973, my father moved out, and my two siblings and I lived with our mother. Two years later, she left. I was eight years old. That's when all three of us were smashed—at six, eight, and eleven years old.

We had just come home from visiting our father at his urban apartment in Massachusetts for the weekend. My mother's parents and her sister were sitting on the couch in the living room. When I heard the news, I sprung forward from where I stood inside the front entrance of the house to the green rotary-dial telephone sitting on the cherry-wood table five feet ahead of me. I picked up the receiver, the tangled chord unraveling, and jammed my finger into the hole with the letters ABC affixed above it. I turned the wheel hard and fast, my hand trembling, my entire body trembling. But I did not cry. My sister sobbed and ran up to her bedroom. I don't remember how my brother reacted. Because I didn't know what else to do, I continued dialing, as if I knew where to find my mother. If she answered the phone, she'd hear my small voice telling her how sorry I was for whatever I had done wrong. She'd come right home and we'd start all over again, as if she had never left. I kept waiting for the sound of her voice. But, of course, she never answered the phone. All I heard was a piercing pitch indicating a misdialed number.

After my mother left, a long-time family friend moved in with my siblings and me while our father lived in his apartment and began searching for a house large enough for three kids.

A month passed before I saw my mother again at her apartment in Cambridge, Massachusetts. Sitting cross-legged on her bed, my eyes explored the cramped room: blank walls, chipped wooden dresser, a single window stained with the city's pollution. I don't remember what we talked about; I was the "quiet" child she would come to describe me as. Quiet, and afraid.

A couple of years after I moved to Vermont, while my mother was visiting me in Montpelier, we reminisced about when I was a kid and how my younger cousin and I would crawl under my grandmother's coffee table to devour a candy-dish bowl of miniature Reese's Peanut Butter Cups, as if we couldn't be seen beneath the glass top. Such reminiscing led my mother to prod me, not for the first time, about having children. "You'll regret it if you don't. What will you do when you're eighty and you don't have children to help or visit you?"

I had already told her, more than once, that I liked my freedom, and had no intention of having children. I hadn't told her she was part of the real reason, nor did I ask the question I had refrained from asking for years, because I didn't know how to phrase it without hurting her. But this time, a spell of courage drove me to ask: "Mom, what was it that made you leave?"

Her chest heaved and her eyes welled up. She turned away from me, away from my question, and looked out the window at autumn painting the woods like a watercolor.

In that moment, a part of me wished I could have taken my question back.

She looked back at me, wiping a tear. "I couldn't take care of you kids."

I raised a brow at her. I recalled the nights before she left, when she would shake my bedcovers to scare the boogeyman away; the time she rushed my brother to the emergency room after he climbed onto a closet shelf and fell, his teeth breaking through his tongue; then another trip to the ER after he ate mothballs off the neighbor's lawn. My mother could have taken care of us, I thought.

"I didn't have the money," she said. She had worked part-time as a journalist at a local television station while my father ran his full-time business as a real estate developer.

It wasn't enough of an answer for either of us, and I still didn't get it, but seeing her deeply troubled expression, I didn't push.

"Your father . . ." she paused. "He hit me." She looked down, playing with the wad of tissue in her hand. "He wouldn't give me enough money, even when we were married. When I was on my own, I had to beg him for it, but I was afraid. I knew if I left, he'd have the money to take care of you kids."

Listening to her, I saw myself at seven years old, watching my mother standing on the front steps of the house. My father is angrily shoving a check at her. He barges down the steps and back to the car. She yells out to him, something about it not being enough. He turns, pointing a finger at her, screams, "You're not getting another dime." I scurry toward the edge of the driveway, my fingers plugging my ears.

"Leaving was the only option I had," my mother continued. She dabbed the mascara streaking her cheek. "Melissa, I hope you know how sorry I am, so, so sorry that I hurt you kids. I never wanted to hurt you. I just didn't know what else to do."

I didn't ask her why she didn't seek help from her parents, friends, or a therapist. I didn't think the answer would have been enough for the little girl I was, but the woman I had become did not press her for more answers. Both the little girl and I needed more love, but both of us remained quiet.

Sitting in my wheelchair here at Cedars, the matzo ball soup now cold, I wish I said "yes" when my mother turned toward me one more time before leaving Cedars for the East Coast and said, "Maybe I should stay."

My father's physical abuse toward me and my siblings started after we moved in with him. He bloodied my brother's face when he was twelve. My father was driving us somewhere when, from the back seat, I saw him strike my brother in the nose. I remember curling up against the door, choking back a whimper before it could escape. I don't remember what my brother did to deserve a fist in the face.

When I was thirteen, he chased me from the kitchen, through the living room, into my bedroom, screaming, "You listen to me. Right now."

I cowered in the corner of the room, both hands over my face, shaking, holding my breath. Inches from him, my sharp, ice-skating scribe was leaning against the wall. He grabbed it, and pointed the metal tip over my head.

"Look at me!" he yelled.

"I'm sorry, I'm sorry," I cried, peeking through my fingers at my father's clenched jaw, spittle forming at the corners of his mouth. In between sobs, I promised I would not do whatever it was I had done wrong again. Had I forgotten to take out the trash, empty the dishwasher, feed the dog?

Hearing my mother's story about why she had left, I wondered if she had considered that my father might abuse my siblings and me. Still, I didn't want to ask her. If she had considered his potential violence towards his children, then the next logical question would be a repeat of the first. "What was it that made you leave?"

I wondered if my father was also incapable of caring for three children. Like my mother, maybe he wasn't prepared. I never asked him if he regretted marrying in his early twenties, or about the divorce. The one time I dared to ask him why he never talked about what drove him to hit us, he said, in a brittle, somewhat sad voice, "I'm sorry," followed-up with, "But that's the past. Let's talk about good things."

—

I'm in the hospital at LA General, my father sits by the window near my bed, reading *USA Today.* A shrewd businessman, he likes to keep abreast of the latest interest rates and numbers of new homes being built. He pulls a yellow pad out of his briefcase. I shake off the narcotic nap and turn to face the sun pouring through the window. I spy a golden shimmer off the pad's edges, the sun shining on my father's bald spot as he leans into the page, urgently scribbling something. He stops to rub his chin, as though he's contemplating a financial transaction, or thinking about all the work he has left behind at home. I wonder if he feels inconvenienced for having to fly all the way from Florida to California, and on such brief notice.

With each passing day, the pages of my father's pad furl, like late October leaves. When deliberating over his notes, the shallow wrinkles in his forehead deepen, so deep I envision my own curiosities crawling inside them: *Dad, what are you writing?* If he remembers something important, he mutters to himself, "I need to call Jack. His loan payment is due next week." As he hurriedly scratches the reminder on his pad, I close my eyes and fall back asleep. He keeps a pen close at all times, usually in the side pocket of his Dockers. For as long as I can recall, my father has had a knobby protrusion on his middle finger from all the pen gripping.

When the doctors give me permission to go outside without a medical professional, my father puts aside his pad and pen to join me. He pushes me to the front entrance of LA General, where I hunker in the wheelchair, wearing a sack-like gown. With a starched blanket wrapped around my torso, I tilt my head toward the full sun, my anemic face and chilled nose feeling every particle of warmth. Not ten minutes into our outing, a middle-aged woman stops in front of us and says, "It looks like you've been banged up quite a bit."

I startle at her voice and nearly slingshot out of my chair. *What makes you think that?* I want to say. *Oh, right, the wheelchair, the cast, and the bruises are all dead giveaways.* Thank God, the sarcasm is quickly pre-empted by my brain's empathy circuitry, and I get that she's speaking from a position of compassion.

I respond to the woman with a quick smile, then spread the bottom half of the blanket over the cast, and the rest up around my arms, camouflaging my wounds and bruises. As for the Rorschach bruise surrounding my left eye and temple, I'll need a lot of makeup to hide that brown blot.

The woman smiles in return and continues toward the hospital entrance, leaving behind a cloud of perfume.

"I'm tired," I tell my father. "Let's go back inside."

"Are you sure?" he asks, hoisting up his high-waisted khakis. "It's really nice out. I like being around people."

"I want to go back to bed."

Before he leaves to return to the East Coast, the day after I am transferred to Cedars, my father hands me a copy of an English translation of a Hebrew blessing. "I read this every time I get on a plane," he says. "It's a journey blessing."

As a drifted Jew, prayer has never been a part of my travel or daily routine, other than when I studied for my Bat Mitzvah. Except for the Jewish High Holy Days, my family rarely attended Temple. And we celebrated Passover mostly for the food. When observing the holiday with my father, we had baked brisket, salted matzo, and kugel, a sweet egg-noodle casserole. When my mother took us to her parents on the second day of Passover, we ate the same foods again, with the added treat of my grandmother's homemade tzimmes, a sugary stew of carrots, sweet potatoes, and dried fruits. My Judaism was never about prayer.

My father always acted with extra caution; he unplugged the toaster and shut off the water before leaving for a weekend getaway, obsessions born of his childhood burn trauma. But until he gave me the copy of the blessing, I didn't know he relied on prayer to feel safe. He attended High Holy Days services at Brandeis University, but, as he often said, "I go because I like the music." He also kept a prayer book, *The Gates of Heaven*, by his bed. Sometimes he brought it with him to the breakfast table.

He'd rest one hand on the closed prayer book while jotting notes on his yellow pad. If I were close enough to the pad, I'd peek at his scrawl: "Call realtor about new land for sale ... purchase more life insurance ... check CD rates." Maybe the prayer book was a talisman of sorts for my father. Maybe by laying his hand on the cover, he believed a prayer could seep its way into him and deliver a solution to whatever it was he was working through in his mind. In some ways, he was a simple man. The type of person who would put a history book under his pillow instead of studying for the exam. Because of all the scraps of paper he kept in it, all the reminders scratched in blue ink, the spine of the prayer book was worn and stretched. At one point, he had to Scotch tape it back together. I always thought it was odd that he stored his business and financial strategies in a prayer book. But maybe he believed the closer his strategies were to prayer, the greater the chance he'd be successful. Now, knowing all this about my father, I wonder in what other ways he relied on prayer.

As soon as he leaves my hospital room, I unfold the blessing and read it. "Now that I begin a new journey, I turn to You in confidence and trust. May I go forth in health and safely reach my destination. May this journey not be in vain; let its purpose be fulfilled." I would read it again on my flight back to the East Coast a week later.

But, for now, I need to find a secure place to keep the blessing. Like my father, who tucked notes inside his prayer book, I tuck it between the pages of *The Secret Life of Bees*, where Lily's curiosity, determination, and fearlessness working with bees help her to conquer her traumas: her father's abuse and her accidental shooting of her mother. Ultimately, she reinvents herself.

I forgot that Lily's middle name is Melissa, and that she grew up on a peach farm.

Part II

Chapter 17

Entering Vermont. The modest green sign welcomes me back home. It's August 6, three weeks since the peach flew out of my hand. My mother picks me up at the airport in Boston, and we head north to Montpelier. For the next few months, I will be living with my landlords and close friends, Kathleen and Rick, whom I've known since I moved to Vermont over three years ago. As we cross the Connecticut River into Vermont, my mother driving, and me in the back with my legs stretched across the seat, I place my cheek against the window's smooth glass and gaze up into the wide-open sky. I wonder what it would be like to swim, limber and weightless, in all that borderless blue. I roll down the window, stick my head out, let the wind whoosh in my ears and my long hair billow behind me like the tail of a kite. I admire the river's patient, meandering flow; its peaceful presence is a meditation.

As my mother pulls up the steep hill and into the driveway of Kathleen and Rick's home, I inhale Vermont—herbs, berries, hay. Kathleen, Rick, and their two children, fourteen-year-old Ainsley and twelve-year-old Ben, are waiting for us at the top of the driveway. Rick stands between Ainsley and Ben, all three of them wearing steady smiles, as if they are posing for a family portrait. I open the car door, and their dog Baxter runs up to me, panting into the early August humidity, his tail wagging like a windshield wiper on high speed. A youthful forty-three-year-old, Kathleen wears familiar summer attire: a bouquet-printed sundress, Teva sandals, and a yellow bandana to hold her hair back. Her cheeks are flushed, as if she has been outside working in the sunny garden. Wearing a cotton dress shirt with the sleeves rolled up, Rick looks like he has just come home from his office at his architecture firm. As my mother learned from watching the physical therapists at the hospital maneuver my wheelchair, she lines it up parallel to the back seat of the car. Beyond that, she knows not to interfere, avoiding another, "Please, let me do it."

With Kathleen, Rick, and the kids nervously watching, I lift myself up with my arms, plant my butt in the chair, and swing my legs over, all in one smooth sweeping motion. The movement scares Rick, who calls out, "Whoah." I look up at him with his mouth agape, as if he's bracing himself for the upside-down flip on a roller coaster.

"Welcome back!" Kathleen cheers.

—

"Check out the wheelchair ramp," Ben says. "My dad and I found some old wood out back and built it for you." His eyes, as blue as his father's, sparkle like a sun-flecked lake.

A lump forms in my throat, but I won't let myself cry, not in front of Ben. Instead, I give him a half smile and wheel over the weathered plank leading from the garage into the kitchen. The plank thumps, like when a car drives over a rickety wooden bridge and you ready yourself for the collapse.

"Cool," Ben says. "Dad, it works."

I wheel into the dining room off the kitchen. Kathleen and Rick have transformed it into a bedroom: single bed, nightstand, dresser. The hardwood floors shine and smell clean, natural, like Murphy's Pure Vegetable Oil Soap.

Kathleen opens a dresser drawer. "See, there's lots of room for your clothes." She spins around, takes three brisk strides to the narrow closet in the corner, and opens the door. "You can put your clothes in here, too." Dry dust drifts out. I sneeze.

"That looks familiar." I point to the white commode at the end of the bed.

"I got it from the Center for Independent Living," Kathleen says. "I've got a Costco-size bottle of Lysol to go with it." My mother erupts in laughter. I force a chuckle and smile at Kathleen. I'm thinking about the fluorescent blaze of chemical yellow, the world I discovered when the psychologist at Cedars explained survivor's guilt.

"We're glad you're staying with us," Kathleen says. I press my teeth together, holding back a grumble. I want to be at my apartment, taking care of myself. But it makes sense to stay with Kathleen and her family. The apartment I had rented from them three years earlier is on the second floor, and the bedroom on the third.

Kathleen thrives on helping others. She isn't only a mother, but also a professional caretaker. She feeds babies at a daycare center, changes their diapers, coddles crying toddlers with bloody knees and noses, and tenderly places cool cloths on the foreheads of feverish children. Despite my yearning to be back at my apartment, I am grateful for Kathleen and Rick's outpouring of support.

A curtain of purple flowers, a virtual garden, separates the living room from my temporary bedroom. As I wheel close to it, it flaps like the jib of a sailboat. The curtain is penetrable to all sounds, even the most private ones. But at least the heavy cotton prevents anyone from seeing through. Me on one side. Everyone else on the other side.

Sometimes I prefer it that way, to be on one side, beyond others' view. Behind the curtain is where I give myself permission to listen to my avalanching thoughts and try to make sense of them. Or I curl up under the sheets and fall asleep, my attempt at taking a break from the accident. Along with the bed, the small ex-dining room holds the wheelchair, the commode, and is decorated with the calendar hanging above the bed, most of the squares filled in with medical appointments or physical therapy sessions. When no one is home, and I know I can't be heard, I lie on the bed with the curtain closed and cry until I'm too tired to cry any longer. Once in a while, I even give myself permission to speak "I hate you" with abandon to the wall or ceiling. But on the other side of the curtain, in earshot of others, I am "the quiet one," easygoing, agreeable, always wearing a big smile.

Chapter 18

"Do you like the bed next to the window?" Kathleen asks. "You'll be able to watch the chickens." Through dust pixels, I gaze out at the yard from a distance. A few chickens scamper through the grass, pecking at each blade. Though I've lived in Montpelier for more than three years, and have eaten eggs laid by Kathleen and Rick's chickens, everything, even the chickens, seems new to me. It was only two days ago when I peered through the hospital window at Cedars into a world of traffic, concrete, and smog.

I roll up to the bed, where a bulging manila envelope lies, pull open the clasp, and dump the sealed get-well cards—yellows, pinks, blues, and greens—onto the quilt. I recognize some of the handwriting on the envelopes: a coworker's calligraphy, a friend's curlicue M, a neighbor's accomplished cursive. So many unique Melissas. Randomly, I pick up a card, turn it over, slide my finger beneath the sealed flap. I stop. Quickly, I gather the unopened cards, tuck them back into the manila envelope. *Later. Another time. Too many.* I can't decide which Melissa to choose. Do I want the one that resembles the woman I've always known: the accomplished cursive for the perfectionist Melissa, or the curlicue M and calligraphy for the playful Melissa?

My father sends me Hallmark cards. "Love yourself, make peace with who you are at this moment. Try. Take chances. The next rock in your path may be a stepping-stone." When he visited me at Cedars, I believed he didn't know how to help me in the way I needed helping—by listening and encouraging me to explore. But when I read his cards, I wonder if he chose them with conscious intent, as an encouragement for me to explore. Or maybe he plucked them from a store shelf in a hurry before heading to his office, unaware of what those words would come to mean to me. Did he know that I'd become wary of taking chances, that it would be a long time before I found that next rock, that I'd continue to have to work hard at loving myself? I never thought to ask my father those questions before he slipped into the fog of Alzheimer's.

Kathleen picks up my pillow and fluffs it. "I thought you'd want your own." I smile and forget about the heap of cards. For years, I slept on that same pillow each night, my head busy with bad dreams about work: dropping a preemie, forgetting to feed a baby, injecting too much medication into a baby's IV. Somehow, I slept through them. Now, traumatic dreams of a different sort violate my sleep. A car accelerating toward me. A mother screaming for someone to help her baby. Bodies smacking into a car windshield. I run my hand across the bedsheets warmed by the sun's rays. The scent of fabric softener prevails over the wet August air.

The eight-by-ten photograph I took years ago of a bicycle hangs on the wall above the head of the bed. Kathleen chose that one to decorate my room. *Hmm... She knows me well, but I don't think I've ever told Kathleen it's one of my favorites.* In the photo, the rusted bicycle hangs by chains on the outside wall of a ramshackle antique shop. Dried vines, thick as ropes, wrap themselves around the seat and center shaft. The bike is old, tired. A short two months earlier I was biking with a friend through the dense woods of Stowe. My feet locked into the pedals, I hopped over logs, pedaled through streams, letting the cool water and mud splash my legs. Getting dirty was proof of hard exercise. Now, I wonder when, or if, I'll ride my mountain bike again. Because I was in top physical condition before the accident, the surgeons assured me that I'd return to the activities I once enjoyed. But I worry that my legs have been still for too long. If they don't move soon, in the way that I've trained them—fast and vigorous—they'll become stiff and rusty.

That evening, we all gather on the front porch for a barbecue. The sun descends over the Worcester Range like a red hot-air balloon. I squint, trying to home in on Mount Hunger, twelve miles away, where I have hiked numerous times. Oh, how much I want to touch its open-faced peak, each crag, each moss-covered rock, each marble-smooth boulder.

That first night back in Vermont, the nightmares begin. They downpour on my sleep like an unexpected weather front. No advisories. No warnings.

> *The driver loses control of the wheel. I grip the passenger-side door handle. We veer off the road and over a cliff. The car rolls upside down, plummets hundreds of feet into a gray canyon, my stomach dropping and twisting. I try to scream, but it won't come out.*

> *Someone is driving a car. It flies up into the air, smashes to the ground, rolls onto its side, glass shattering. It rolls again, toward me. I run, faster, faster....*

I wake, clenching my sweat-soaked t-shirt, my chest burning. Several minutes later, after my chest muscles relax and a subdued breathing pattern returns, I turn over the pillow under my head, the one Kathleen brought from my apartment. With the cool side now soft against my cheek, I feel comforted to be living with good friends. I know they are in bed one flight above me, and Baxter is lying a few feet away, just beyond the purple-flowered curtain, his tail steadily sweeping across the floor. Within minutes, the crickets and frogs lull me back into a deep sleep.

Chapter 19

While I thrash in bed at night from the nightmares, trying to convince myself that they are not real and cannot hurt me, others endure the fallout of the crash, too. Jenna, a budding actress, who was shopping for oranges when the Buick careened through the market, remembers being pinned to the ground by a flying table. She suffers from PTSD so debilitating she experiences "thrashing" flashbacks, stutters, and can't read or recall simple words. For eight months after the accident, she will not be able to sleep or stop crying. She ends up having to be treated in a psychiatric unit.

Shamsi's dreams: the Buick is coming at her snakelike; it strikes her and wraps her around the tree. She slides down and feels the back of her head whack the ground.

Sandra's dreams: she's lying flat on the pavement, looking up at the clouds while news helicopters circle the scene. She sees "the carnage of humanity painting blood on concrete."

"Carnage." That word again. The same word Tina used to describe the war-like scene at the market. Not dream carnage. Wide-awake carnage.

In December 2016, a failed asylum seeker hijacked a truck and drove it through a crowd of shoppers strolling through a popular market in Berlin. In December 2024, a right-wing extremist physician from Saudi Arabia drove a rented car through a market in Magdeburg. In October 2017, another terrorist plowed a rented van into dozens of joggers and bicyclists on a path along the Hudson River in New York City, leaving a seventeen-block trail of scattered bodies and crumpled bikes.

These attacks were undeniably and sickeningly familiar to those of us who had experienced wide-awake carnage on that fateful day in Santa Monica. Unlike Russell Weller, the terrorists who struck in Germany and New York were homicidal in their impulses and planning. But the wholesale destruction was the same, the traumatic recollections eerily alike. "Boom, boom," survivors heard in New York. A "massive bang" in Berlin, Germany. In Magdeburg, "the aftermath resembled a warzone."

I try breathing deeply and slowly when I wake from my nightmares. When that doesn't calm me, I practice the visualization technique I learned from a psychologist who visits me weekly at Kathleen and Rick's home. I close my eyes and picture pleasant images, like butterflies, their orange-and-black wings fluttering with the grace of a ballerina. Other times, wildflowers bloom behind my twitching eyelids. They sway right to left, left to right, as if a breeze is rocking them to sleep. Occasionally it works; more often, I simply endure.

Each time I wake with a start, my internal screams still echoing in my chest, I am sure others hear them—they are that loud. But when I ask Kathleen and Rick one morning, they say no. They can't hear me. Is anyone hearing the night screams of the others who survived? What do the loved ones of those who perished dream about?

Chapter 20

It's the third week in August when a physical therapist guides me over the pool in a Hoyer Lift, an industrial-strength hammock seat attached to a pulley with a crank handle. She inches me lower, lower, toward the turquoise ripples. I stare through them, extending my feet, anticipating the initial dip of my toes in eighty-degree water.

From the pool, another therapist reaches up and guides me out of the hammock. She holds me afloat, cradling me like an infant. The first therapist jumps in, and they both support me in their arms, carrying me through the open water. I swish my legs in circles, creating miniature whirlpools around my ankles. The warmth from the water seeps into my skin, massaging every out-of-order joint and tendon. The fracture to the short bone behind my left big toe is still healing, and the toe itself pulses in anticipation, as if it is thirsty and has never experienced such relief before. I wiggle all ten toes, spread them apart, flirt with the water, coaxing it to fill each dehydrated space. When I look down at them, they are as pink as orchids.

Both therapists float me into the deep end, where a warm current of water flows around my upper torso. With a belt around my waist to keep me afloat, I cycle my legs slowly. My knees pop with every movement.

"Back and forth," I whisper, swinging my arms in sync with my legs, forming little white foamy peaks. I see myself as a ten-year-old again at summer camp, floating face up in the lake, watching clouds stretch long like melting taffy. I set my eyes on the plaster ceiling, imagine it is the sky, and see those remembered cloud shapes: a duckling, a baby panda, a goldfish. After an hour of pool therapy, my hip joints feel as if they will unhinge from my torso. But my big toe no longer pulses. Even the discs between my vertebrae feel as if they have been lubricated, the fibrous tissues now flexible and elastic, as they should be.

I want to live in the turquoise ripples, making skiing motions, circling my arms, creating a white froth. I want to float on my back, my arms and legs and fingers and toes stretched wide, play in my personal playground until I'm able to walk again. Another ten weeks, at least.

As much as I want to float forever in this blue bath, I still have a lot more work to do. A physical therapist centers a toy rubber pig over my stomach. It smells like Play-Doh. "Take a deep breath and slowly exhale," she says. "It's important to think about your breathing." She reminds me that I'm at risk of developing pneumonia due to my fractured ribs. And being sedentary—spending much of the day sitting in the wheelchair, if not in bed—doesn't help. Because I'm a nurse, I know the risks, but think I'm already breathing deeply enough.

I inhale, my stomach rounding into a second-trimester bulge, the pig itself bulging—an eerie illusion, like a sculpted, outie belly button. I let all the air out, and puff up my belly again, the pig wobbling like a drunken sow. After a few breaths, I feel as if I am working against enormous pressure. Pain jabs my diaphragm. Maybe it's gas. Either that, or I am constipated, which shouldn't come as a surprise, given all the Vicodin I've been taking. The physical therapist offers a better explanation.

"You've been guarding yourself against the pain," she says. Which means I haven't been taking deep enough breaths. I've actually forgotten *how* to breathe effectively. This is the first time since the accident a month ago—or has it been longer?—that I've taken full breaths. I take the pig home, and several times a day, I place it over my belly button, watch it rise then fall, its black-dotted eyes pointing straight at me, as if suspicious I might drag it off to the slaughterhouse. Never. No way. Or, as the expression goes, "In a pig's eye."

I eventually lose the pig, and have to remind myself to take deep breaths, to keep pushing against a puzzling pressure, a pressure I'll be able to name after lots of therapy. Repressed anger and frustration. I am angry and frustrated because I'm tired of fear as my go-to emotion. I'm angry and frustrated—and afraid—that the fear itself will thwart my motivation to be more than I am. But first, I have to define who I am. How do you name yourself when your identity has been defined as a nurse for twenty years? It's like a tattoo; once it's etched into your skin, it's with you for the rest of your life.

Russell Weller's identity tattoo is changing shape. A retired food-sales broker and Korean War veteran, he is hospitalized three times after the accident for cardiac issues and an infection. He is no longer the outgoing man his neighbors and family describe him as, the man who once welcomed guests into his home, who hosted holiday dinners, tutored high school students, and organized book sales for his local library. A father figure who taught his nephew how to use a hammer, knot a tie, and throw a ball, he now keeps the door to his house closed and the window shades drawn. He manages to care for his wife, who is also ill, making her coffee and sandwiches each day. But he rarely leaves the home they've lived in for fifty-two years, not even for groceries. He has them delivered. Russell Weller has essentially become a recluse.

I will walk in ten weeks. My breathing will become stronger. I will create a new identity tattoo. What does the tattoo of a recluse even look like?

Chapter 21

Sitting in the wheelchair, I see myself as idle, and that old demon from my youth returns to haunt me. I'm afraid I'll gain weight, too much weight. I've been given a second go at life, another round in the ring, and here I am letting my phobia of putting on pounds take up healing space. I'm forgetting about the number of calories I am burning while pressing the plates of the Total Gym, or while kicking and cycling my legs in the pool.

My mother drives four hours from Massachusetts, taking time off from her demanding work as a marketing consultant; she wants to see for herself that I'm eating. "Melissa, it scares me when you don't eat," she says, while making me breakfast one morning at Kathleen and Rick's. For her sake, I nibble on a slice of dry toast topped with a fried egg.

As much as her quintessential Jewish worry makes me roll my eyes, I recognize her steady stare, the stare that says she is afraid I'll regress to my high school days, when miniskirts were the hottest trend and Tab was the nourishment of choice among young girls. I was seventeen when I started starving myself. As my weight plummeted, neither one of my parents noticed at first. At the time, I was living with my father, and the ice cream store he had recently opened commanded much of his attention. As for my mother, my siblings and I saw her mostly on weekends, when she'd take us to visit our grandparents, who also hadn't noticed my weight loss, or at least didn't say anything if they had. When my father and I were out for Chinese food one evening, and I reluctantly poked my fork into a piece of steamed broccoli like it was burdock while he feasted on fried rice and pork strips, I couldn't hold back any longer. "Dad, you know, I've lost twenty-five pounds." I was proud of myself for losing the weight, and hoped he'd be proud of me, too.

He stopped chewing, and dropped his fork on the plate, the tines clanking against the porcelain. "Whoa. Why did you lose so much weight?"

"I just did." I didn't know what else to say. All I could think about was his question, which I translated into, "What's wrong with you?"

I continued to drop weight, until my bony face floated above my loose sweaters and baggy jeans. My father moved from curiosity to alarm, and he made an appointment with my pediatrician. The doctor diagnosed me with anorexia nervosa and referred me to a nutritionist. She taught me how to count calories, so calories I counted, every single painful one. I battled back against my best interest. At dinnertime I'd make excuses as to why I couldn't eat: a stomachache, too much homework, too tired. My easily frustrated father would quickly lose his patience. "Come out of that room! You're going to fucking eat!" As usual, my father coped with his helplessness through anger. But all it did was drive me to continue starving myself. The more weight I lost, the more in control I felt, not only in control of my body, but also in control of my own choices. No one could stop me. My mother read book after book about anorexia and told me she was afraid I was going to die. I lost forty pounds within seven months.

When I could barely stand up on my own, my father called the pediatrician in a panic. He told my father to immediately get me to the hospital. I had to be stopped. I had reached a perilous point. I was headed for death.

I spent ten days in the hospital, the time it took for nurses and doctors to equilibrate my out-of-whack internal chemistry with IV fluids and electrolyte supplements. I was discharged under the condition that I continue treatment with a psychiatrist, which, for the next four years, I did. During that time, I learned to eat healthfully, and slowly gained enough weight to keep me away from a return trip to the hospital. By the time I graduated college, I believed I had been cured. Eventually, I even granted myself moments of indulgence: a few bites of dark chocolate or a scoop of Ben and Jerry's Cherry Garcia ice cream.

Yes, I understood my mother's look when she said, "It scares me when you don't eat."

While using the wheelchair, I feel little control over my body, and though it's been years since counting calories has become an ordinary part of my day-to-day life, as routine as brushing my teeth, I still approach eating like a guard at a castle gate, screening all foods before granting them entry into my body.

Without realizing it, eating becomes an act—more to please others than to please myself—and I start in with the old script. "That's too spicy," or "That upsets my stomach." Patty, a close friend, visits me at Kathleen and Rick's with high-calorie shakes made with organic peanut butter, flaxseed oil, soy milk, and protein powder. Knowing her, I'm certain she has put time and effort into shopping for the best ingredients for those shakes. The shakes are probably pretty tasty, but I'm suspicious of calories that cannot be easily counted, and I convince myself that the texture of the shakes is a lot like sand. I slurp down a few sips then leave the shake on the bedside table. Once it curdles, I pour it down the kitchen sink drain. I throw away vitamins, amino acids, healthful fats—nourishment for the body. I am lying to myself that I have been cured.

After my mother returns to Massachusetts, my cellphone chimes with a call from her every morning, a big change from our casual Sunday check-ins before the accident. "Did you have breakfast?" she asks. "What did you eat? Have you had lunch yet? Why not?" She suggests I eat high protein foods like tuna fish or cheese. "Great ideas, Mom," I say, hoping to appease her. "I've got this." When she visits me, she runs her hands over my papery arms, and says, "You still look too skinny. I don't think you've been eating enough. Let me make you lunch. I'm your mother." Which I understand to mean, "I need another chance at being your mother again." But I don't want my mother to feed me as she did during the initial days of my hospitalization, when she thought I liked large doses of lemon Jell-O. I will not give up control of my body to anyone.

The math is all that matters. An excess number of calories in and too few calories burned equals weight gain. But while at physical therapy one day, the therapist shares something startling. "You need one hundred grams of protein a day." I slap my hand over my mouth. I know the recommended daily allowance for adult women is around forty-five grams. "Your body is healing," she says, "and you're burning a lot of energy getting around in the wheelchair." She suggests I eat eggs to achieve one hundred grams. I look up a protein table online and calculate the math in my head. *Six grams of protein in an egg. One hundred divided by six equals sixteen eggs! At that rate, I'll turn into an egg. And at eighty calories per egg, that's over thirteen hundred calories. Fuck that!* Instead, I choose prepared foods, like Pure Protein bars, which are clearly labeled with nutritional facts: thirty-one grams of protein, three hundred calories per bar. Washed down with eight ounces of skim milk—eight grams of protein—I fulfill almost half my required protein intake for the day. The bars allow me to reach the one-hundred-gram goal, while avoiding stuffing myself with a truckload of calories.

I had to be scared into believing I needed more calories.

During an appointment with an orthopedic surgeon, she points at a lit-up screen with an x-ray of my healing foot. "You have osteopenia." She doesn't need to explain, because she knows I know. Softening of the bones. All the sitting, along with no weight-bearing exercise, poses a risk for osteopenia. "I know about your history of anorexia," she says. I tilt my head at her, wondering how she knows; I haven't said a word to her about my past. And why would she bring up something that happened such a long time ago? I'm convinced anorexia no longer holds sway over me, but how wrong I am. It's still wedged in the present. Anorexia is still with me—a faded scar, but with palpable edges.

"Anorexia causes lasting damage," she says, "not just osteoporosis." She looks at my fingers. That's how she knows. The blue discoloration, a sign of poor circulation—Raynaud's Phenomenon, brought on by low body weight. "You need to eat more, for bone health."

I stare at my foot's skeleton fixed in black-and-white on the x-ray screen. The bones remind me of matchsticks. I wrap my numb fingers around my skinny wrist and push on the splinter-like bones, feeling them wiggle back and forth. *What if I turn into my grandmother?* She suffered from osteoporosis—porous bones –a risk factor for fractures. In her later years, she walked hunched forward like a bent tree.

Chapter 22

Feeling my thinning bones shift inside of me, I remember the fifteen-year-old girl with anorexia I cared for at Boston Children's Hospital eighteen years ago. I was a new nurse, a year out of college, a year after completing outpatient treatment for anorexia. The other nurses didn't know about my history of an eating disorder. Nor did the teenager. My privacy was my privacy. And for nurses to share their personal struggles was tantamount to crossing professional boundaries. If I had told the teenager about my own battle with anorexia, I'd risk sounding like a victim. As a healthcare professional, I knew priority number one was to look out for her best interests, which meant shoving aside my own demons to make space for hers.

Because her blood pressure and heart rate were initially too low, she had to remain on bed rest. She tucked herself beneath the starched sheets, usually facing the windows, the shades drawn. She was as pale as wax, and the long ends of her brown hair were dry and faded, like withered grass. I rarely saw her smile, and she never looked at me, but in front of me, or behind me. When I walked into her room each day with a "Good morning," she'd nod or mumble. If I asked her how she slept the night before, she'd shrug her shoulders and say, "I guess okay." Perhaps her responses were normal for a teenager. But I also knew she was angry with me, with all the nurses who cared for her, because we subjected her to an anorexia protocol, the same one the nurses had followed with me. After each meal, patients had to remain on bed rest for an hour. If they didn't finish a meal within thirty minutes, Ensure, a high-calorie liquid supplement, would be offered. Patients were given twenty minutes to drink it, under direct supervision. If they refused to finish the Ensure within the allotted time frame, it would be administered through a nasogastric tube. A weight gain of a quarter pound was expected each day. If patients did not achieve that goal, they had to drink two cans of the Ensure. The protocol was non-negotiable.

When the teenage girl's vital signs stabilized, the nurses allowed "room rest," which meant she was permitted to get out of bed, but could not leave the room. When she used the bathroom, a nurse stood by to make sure she didn't purge or sneak a few minutes of exercise. I'd wait near the bathroom, the door ajar, and listen to her pee into a plastic hat used to measure "output." One time, as she brushed past me on the way into the bathroom, she rolled her eyes at me.

"Sorry," I said, "but you know I have to keep the door open."

"Yep."

When she walked out of the bathroom, she brushed past me as if I wasn't there, back to her bed, back beneath the sheets.

During the week the teenage girl was hospitalized, I wish I had taken the time to ask her what was on her mind, to give her a chance to share her worry about eating and gaining weight. I wish I had realized enough at the time to tell her it was okay for her to be angry, or how I loathed the idea of others having that much control over my body. Or how out of control I truly was when I lost the forty pounds in the first place.

Weighing her each morning while she stood with her back to the scale, so she couldn't see the numbers increase, I'd feel a twinge of envy. *I must weigh a good thirty pounds more than her.* One day, when I counted her caloric intake for breakfast and lunch—a total of seven hundred—I worried that I had overeaten. Yogurt with fruit for breakfast, a turkey sandwich with mustard, and ten pretzel sticks for lunch.

—

I know both the orthopedic surgeon and my mother are looking out for my best interest when they press me to eat. The nurse who sat next to me on my bed eighteen years ago makes an appearance in my mind. I recall how she quietly sat with me while I said, "I don't want to eat… I can't stand being here in this bed, using a commode to pee in… I want to go for a walk… I want to take a shower without people watching me." She kindly allowed me to be angry.

Chapter 23

Alone in my curtained room, I Google "Santa Monica Farmers' Market." In bold Arial font, the words beam from the computer. "Car plows through crowd." Below that is a snapshot of Russell Weller's Buick, the front-end smashed in. An adult body lies nearby, beneath a white tarp, its pale hand and sandaled feet protruding. Next to the body is an open first-aid kit, its contents strewn along a rutted section of Arizona Avenue, as if someone had thrown it aside in a state of helpless rage. A rescue worker steps past the limp body, his head hanging low, his black boot lifted in midstride, hovering over its shadow blackening the already damp pavement. My eyes flit back and forth from the dead body to the distressed rescue worker. My heart fibrillating, my body suddenly feels heavy and I start sweating. My fingers and toes lose sensation, their nails turning the same thunderstorm blue as my bruised feet. It seems my body itself has remembered something from the accident. With a jittery finger-tap of the mouse, I direct the arrow on the screen toward the X icon. Click. Screen closed.

Later that day, I tell Kathleen and Rick I had looked at the photo. "Are you okay?" Rick asks. Kathleen asks me what I saw.

As I describe the photo, she embraces me, and I sink into her fleece pullover, into the aroma of line-dried laundry.

"If it was me, I couldn't look," Rick says.

I don't know how I did it, why I did it. Maybe I needed to witness the loss.

My body's reaction to the photos reminds me why I will not look at the grim images spanning the front pages of the *Santa Monica Daily Press*, *The Los Angeles Times*, The *New York Times*—pages family and friends recently sent me. I stuffed them into a black binder and tucked it out of sight in the closet of my temporary bedroom.

The psychologist who visits weekly while I live with Kathleen and Rick explains that both my reactions to the photos and my nightmares are symptomatic of post-traumatic stress disorder. "Your brain has been rewired," she says during one of her visits. As a nurse, I know that not only war veterans but also those who have experienced any kind of trauma—rape, natural disasters, and abuse—are at risk of developing PTSD. But somehow, I don't see how PTSD applies to me. I look at her as if she is speaking Yiddish. "Your brain is vulnerable to overstimulation," she says. I imagine flat-headed screws loosely holding together all four lobes of my cerebral cortex, the screws stripped useless from too much environmental torque. She's wrong, I think. Out to lunch wrong. I hit a tree once while skiing out of bounds. I've hiked within ten feet of bears. I floated down the Colorado River one summer and got sucked into an eddy. I continued skiing, hiking, and swimming. I don't have PTSD. Nope. Not me.

But then I remember the orthopedic surgeon's cautionary statement during my appointment with her after I returned to Vermont. "The hard part will come later," she said. Other than to clarify that she meant the emotional part will be difficult, she had said nothing more. She squeezed my knee, as if to say, "You'll soon understand what I mean."

After meeting with my psychologist, "The hard part will come later" replays in my head like a CD on continuous loop. Yes, the trauma will linger, in my body and mind. My physiological reactions to the image of the body, the rescue worker, and the nightmares that started during my first night back in Vermont were only the beginning of the "hard part."

To maintain a yearly tradition, on an eighty-degree August afternoon, Patty and I go to the Champlain Valley Fair. She pushes me in the wheelchair through the dusty fairgrounds, veering around a group of rowdy teenagers waiting in line to ride the bumper cars, past a crowd gawking at bunnies with oversized ears, and around parents and their children pointing at a lithe woman walking across a tightrope. Patty steers the chair with the skillful speed and tactics of a New York City cabbie, in search of kettle corn and Vermont's version of soft serve: maple "creemees." Cotton candy, sausages, and fried onions scent the air. Steam from a nearby burger vendor billows toward us. "Oops, I'm so sorry honey," a woman says as she walks past me and bumps into the wheelchair. *Honey?* I wonder how she would address me if I was standing. Am I being oversensitive? I'm somewhat irked by her comment; I don't even consider how *I* address wheelchair users. Patty backs me up, close to the kettle corn vendor, out of the way of pedestrian traffic. She buys a large box, and I munch, one at a time, savoring the sweet-and-salty, air-popped grains.

The crowd thins, and Patty pushes me forward in the direction of the alpacas. Someone dressed as a robot stands a few feet ahead of us, greeting children as they pass. "Patty, please don't wheel me by him," I plead. (I've always been wary of carnival mascots, uncertain of who's inside.) She pushes me directly past him, her naturally graying curls bouncing as she rolls me over a hump in the dirt. "Hey, nice fish," a male voice speaks, referring to the white sundress patterned with a school of blue fish I borrowed from Kathleen. I tuck my head into my lap and can't help but laugh.

We finally find the vendor selling creemees: vanilla with real Vermont maple syrup. I run my tongue around the top, working my way down to the base, repeating this pattern until all there is left is the melted creemee inside the cone. I tilt my head back and tip the cone into my mouth, slurping down the syrupy vanilla soup. It lasts on my tongue long after we leave. The tickle of sugar.

To help with my recovery, others encourage me to learn a new skill, like how to knit a scarf. "It's relaxing," a friend says one day. Talk about an epic fail. I drop stitches, make holes that look like a swarm of moths have eaten through the yarn, and create knots that not even a contest-worthy knitter can undo. And to keep count—knit one, purl two—forget it. In the end, knitting is literally a pain in the neck. Sometimes I try out new skills on my own. I choose calligraphy, practicing by transcribing music lyrics from some of my favorite artists like Enya's "Ever Close Your Eyes and Listen," or Mary McCaslin's "Looking Back it Makes Me Wonder Where We're Going." I'm good at calligraphy, and so I like it. I begin to see keeping busy as a form of self-preservation. I'm taking my time to face the "hard part."

The September after the fair, Kathleen and Rick take Ainsley, Ben, and me apple picking, my favorite fall activity. As Rick races me along sloping green hills, the chair tilting to the side, I screech, afraid of toppling over and rolling down the hill. He straightens the chair; we laugh so hard my stomach cramps. Once he catches his breath, he runs with me again, through a pocket of cider-donut spiced air. He swerves around downed apples, my body rocking side to side. We laugh some more.

At the back of the orchard, Ben climbs up a tree lush with ripe McIntosh and pitches a few to Ainsley and Kathleen. Rick wheels me close to another tree. Sheltered by a sweet canopy, I reach with the grasper for a round apple. "C'mon, you can get it," Rick says. I lean forward, stretching my arm farther, and poke at the branch. It swings back and forth a few times before I gain a purchase on it. Pulling the branch toward us, I yell for Ben to grab the apple. He gently twists it, snapping it clean off, and holds it out for me. Balancing it in my open palm, I eye the apple for blemishes. None. I roll it along my leg until its skin glimmers, then sink my teeth into the pulp. Tart yet sweet. My gums tingle. The fluids in my body slow, like still lake water. Fall in Vermont is a sweet distraction.

Chapter 24

The placard, labeled "disabled," dangles from the rearview mirror of Rick's car. A red placard. Red for protection, for priority.

He pulls the car into the full parking lot of the restaurant, where we plan to eat lunch with Kathleen and the kids. He drives forward a few more feet, the tires crunching early September leaves, and notices a van parked in the only handicapped accessible space. He parks, blocking the van in. He throws the shifter into park, and with a snap turns the key. Shaking his head in disbelief, he steps out of the car and grabs the wheelchair from the trunk. Kathleen and the kids hesitantly step out of the car. Ben's eyes shoot back and forth from his dad's stiff jaw to me, perched in my chair in the middle of the gravel lot. Ainsley's eyes balloon from her face, as if she is thinking, *Oh no, things are going to get bad.*

"I can't believe someone would do this," Rick says. "Why would someone park here if they don't need the spot?" The Rick I know is a guy with a self-conscious laugh; he exudes patience when painting a watercolor of a wooded landscape, or when cooking meals for his family and me. I've never seen him get angry. As my body curls inward with tension, I whisper to myself, "It's okay, Rick is just looking out for you, Melissa."

We wait a good ten minutes before a middle-aged man in a kilt slips out the back door facing the lot. He plods toward the van, but abruptly stops when he sees the five of us staring at him. Rick's nearly six-foot frame appears taller as he approaches the stunned man now standing a few feet from us. Rick lectures him as he points at me then at the van. The man takes a small step closer and, without looking directly at me, says, "I'm really sorry." I direct my gaze down at the gravel. I'm sure I'm making him feel uncomfortable, a young woman sitting in a wheelchair.

I've seen that look of discomfort many times now. A month earlier, while on the flight from California back to Vermont, two men wheeled me in an aisle chair onto the airplane. Eyes lifted from newspapers to steal a glimpse of me, then quickly shifted back to the page. I knew what the other passengers were wondering, because I wondered the same before my wheelchair days: *What happened to her?* Maybe we ask, or imply, that question—"what happened?"—because we're simply curious. But I also believe we quickly look or walk away from the answer, because we're afraid: *That could be me.* And who wants to be reminded of their own limitations?

A few days after the parking lot incident, while in my wheelchair rolling through downtown Montpelier, I see a thirty-something-year-old guy in an automatic wheelchair motoring toward me. I've seen him in town in the past, and know he can't speak; he communicates with the aid of a keyboard attached to a set of bars jutting out from the front of his chair. "Turn me around now," I say to the friend I'm with. "Let's go back the other way. Hurry." God, I hope he doesn't see me, I whisper. My last awkward meeting with him was nearly two months earlier when I was jogging through town. As I approached him, he slowed down, everything in his body language inviting me to slow down. Wearing a toothy grin, his circling eyes worked to focus on the arc of my long legs. I quickly waved as I passed him, my feet moving faster and faster. He made me feel uncomfortable, as if the reason he uses a wheelchair is contagious and can somehow reach out and grab me.

My friend spins the chair around and speed-walks in the opposite direction. I'm relieved, but feel a little guilty. I consider what I'm feeling, and try to justify my choice. *What if I don't understand him? I'll have to ask him to repeat himself, probably more than once. I could pretend I understand him, but that scares me even more. He'll see it written all over my stupidly forced smile. Melissa, your fear is a bullshit reason for avoiding him.*

Chapter 25

Over Labor Day weekend, my mother and I attend The New World Festival south of Montpelier to listen to live Celtic and Scottish music. Johnny Cunningham, one of the world's greatest Scottish fiddlers, is scheduled to perform. Most of the performances take place in a historic church, the only wheelchair accessible entrance, an antique elevator with a rusted lattice door. It's out of service.

"This is crazy," my mother says.

But I am determined to hear Johnny play. She wheels me down the sidewalk, toward the front of the church, the wheels thumping over cracks. At the front of the church, my mother stops. "There's no way we can get in." There are twelve steps leading to the entrance, and I know I can't tackle this one on my own. I glance around, looking for other wheelchair users, but it appears as if I am the only one. Everyone else is standing; there is no one else at my eye level. I have to arch my neck back to look at anyone. It occurs to me that I have quickly become used to viewing the world from a low-seated position. I've forgotten what it feels like to look at others eye-to-eye.

Hundreds of festival attendees scurry past us up the stairs, some taking them in twos. Flip-flops clack, sneakers squeak, and sandals shuffle. Two plaid-shirted men notice my mother's hands on her hips, and my shit-what-are-we-going-to-do-now grimace. One of them speaks for the other when he says, "We can carry you up."

"Really?" I ask. "Yes, please."

Each holding one side of the chair, they lift me in one swift motion several inches off the ground. I clasp onto the seat of the swinging chair as they effortlessly carry me up all twelve steps. After my mother and I thank them effusively, she pushes me forward toward the entrance. A cluster of people leap aside as if I am a rattlesnake. I'm uneasy with the attention and perhaps misinterpret their reactions as pity.

Ahead of us lay another twelve steps, all jam-packed with hungry-for-Johnny fans. My mother parks the wheelchair at the base of the stairs, and from a distance, we listen to the delicious melodies rising from Johnny's fiddle. I tap my foot lightly against the chair's footrests, in time with jigs, reels, and a Canadian strathspey. I play the air fiddle, pretend to hold the bow with a light grip, like Johnny, my wrist relaxed, my first three fingers close together, my pinky slightly lifted. I close my eyes like I always do while concentrating on learning a new tune, and quietly hum as Johnny's music sweeps past the crowd and into my hungry ear.

My actual fiddle is in its case, leaning in the quiet corner of the front hallway at Kathleen and Rick's. It's been seven weeks since the accident. It's been seven weeks since I've listened to Irish music. Seven weeks since I've played my fiddle. I wonder if my days of making music are over.

But on the ride back to Kathleen and Rick's, I feel a tickle in my belly. It's one of Johnny's tunes, "Darling's Waltz." The playful and seductive notes trill through me like the gentle touch of a lover's hand moving up and down my spine. I make a pact with myself. I'll pick up my fiddle and play it again.

The day after the concert, with "Darling's Waltz" still alive in my ear, I wheel myself up close to the fiddle. A cobweb hangs from the latch like wispy white hair of an old woman. I reach forward for the latch and hoist the case one-handed onto my lap. I blow the cobweb apart with an explosive breath. Like a kid on day one of Hanukkah, I wrench open the zipper and stick my nose into the waist of the fiddle's body. The scent of aged spruce is the inspiration I need. My days of making music are just beginning.

Sitting straight up in the wheelchair, I set the fiddle under my chin and push the bow back and forth across each metal string. They squeal. I tweak the fine tuners, each one creaking from lack of use as I twist it. Back and forth I push the bow, my fingers clumsy along the strings. Despite the flat notes and off rhythms, I play the first polka I learned, recalling what my teacher said during my lessons. "Play a phrase over and over until you can play it without making a mistake. I continue playing the phrase, still unable to get the D note to sound like a D. It screeches like the tortured cat sounds I created when I first learned how to play the fiddle. But I keep playing until the metal string digs into my stinging finger, forming a tender divot.

After a brief rest, I start up again. The floor above me groans. Quick footsteps shake the stairs. The fiddle slips out from beneath my chin. Bow still in hand, I catch it on my lap. "Ben," I call from behind the curtain, "I forgot you were in your room all this time. Could you hear me?"

"You sounded good," his pre-adolescent voice also out of tune.

"You're too sweet."

I sweep my hand along the fiddle's curved back, rubbing the polished finish. The scent of aged spruce rises from the fiddle like a gentle genie.

In September, when a friend lends me her laptop so I can catch up on two months of emails, the subject line of the first message reads, "Off to Californy."

The message is from John, the Irish musician I met three weeks before the accident at a cozy Vermont pub, in a postcard-perfect town where brides-to-be dream of tying the knot.

His email is dated July 16, 2003.

"Have a fun holiday," he wrote.

His second message from July 20: "Melissa, we heard that you were severely injured at the Farmers' Market in Santa Monica. Hope you come home soon, and we get a chance to play music together. We're praying for you. If there's anything we can do, please ask."

A third more recent message, a little cryptic and curious, reads, "Lots to look forward to."

My inbox is full of all kinds of caring messages I want to respond to, so I answer John briefly. "Thanks for thinking of me and, yes, I hope to play music together with you guys."

Chapter 26

The commentator's voice from National Public Radio startles me from an afternoon nap. *Where am I? Home? The hospital? No, at Kathleen and Rick's.* "George Russell Weller has not been charged with a crime." I sit up too fast. The room spins, tilts. "It has been two months since an older driver plowed into a crowd of people at the Farmers' Market in Santa Monica, California. According to police, Weller says he might have mistaken the gas pedal for the brake." I rub my eyes and swing my legs to the side of the bed. The commentator is introducing a broadcast about senior citizens in Southern California "flocking" to drivers' safety classes in the aftermath of the accident. *Good for them.*

"I've been driving for seventy-five years, and I've been careful," says Joe Grotsky, an eighty-nine-year-old guest on the show who has taken the class. "Now it's other people's turn. Let them be careful." *Did he really say what I think he said?* I lean forward, ready to launch myself across the room to the boom box on the floor. For a moment, I have forgotten about the wheelchair. I grab the remote, turn up the volume. Squeezing my hands between my legs, I glare at the radio's solid red light, the source of the old man's arrogance. "I've decided that my reaction time isn't that bad," he says.

I squeeze my hands harder, my fingernails stabbing my palms. A guest journalist on the show, who is interviewing Grotsky, refers to him as "lucky," because his license won't be taken away. He'll maintain his independence. I hurl a pillow toward the radio. When Grotsky says he'll continue to drive the ten miles to visit his family, I grab the pink pig I used for breathing exercises, and whip that across the room, the pig landing snout up, inches from the red light. *Why doesn't he ask his family to pick him up? Why don't they take his car keys, hide them in a lockbox, throw them out?* His indifference hijacks me, and I get overheated with anger toward Russell Weller. I can taste it, as bitter as vinegar. I'm angry with his family, too. Surely, they knew he was not in any shape to be driving. Why didn't they intervene before people died?

Six years later, as a nurse for aging individuals, I meet Judith, and, for the first time since the accident, begin to see trauma with greater empathy for older drivers. An eighty-nine-year-old with emphysema, it takes a Herculean effort for Judith to get out of bed. "I ain't got no legs," she confesses. I'm aware that she still drives, and ask if she feels safe driving. She says she doesn't drive too far, "Just to Walmart sometimes. I can't ask my kids. My son is in Florida, and my daughter is away for two months." Her voice quivers with a pitiful plea. "I'm begging you, please, don't have them take away my car. It's all I have left." Yet, as a nurse and survivor of an older-driver crash, I feel obligated to act, to call her doctor and her family, urge them to do what it takes to get Judith off the road. If I do nothing, then later learn that she was in a car accident and that people were injured or died, I'd hate myself for being a coward, for turning my back on what I've known all along to be the hard truth: that Judith is unfit to drive.

As close as I am to picking up the phone and calling her family, I don't have to. Not long after my visit with Judith, her family takes her car from her. She breaks down crying as she tells me the news during a follow-up wellness visit. "I don't know what I'll do now."

All I can do is listen and remember how alone and incapable I felt six years earlier when I depended on friends and family to drive me to doctor's appointments, physical therapy, the grocery store, the pharmacy. For Judith, though, it isn't temporary. Her driving days are gone forever.

Entombed in our country's poor public transportation system, especially here in Vermont, to have a car is to be self-reliant, capable, free. Judith's freedom now depended on others. But who would those others be? A senior transport van? Uber? Her neighbors? How long would it take before her neighbors got tired of chauffeuring her from one medical appointment to the next? It's a tragedy that taking away one's car is not accompanied by better support—reliable public transportation, more senior shuttles, community networks—for those left stranded. It could not have been easy for her family, but it's still comforting to know that Judith's family did face the hard choice before Judith became another Russell Weller.

Russell Weller's nephew claimed his uncle had suffered a stroke that caused the crash, but medical exams showed no such evidence. He was awake and alert when he sped through the market. Bystanders witnessed his hands on the steering wheel, in the ten-and-two position. And though he had a history of orthopedic conditions, and needed to use a cane on occasion, he otherwise walked and moved without any apparent difficulties.

"Grotsky plans to turn off his car radio to limit distractions," the radio journalist continues with a light humorous tone, "but only after he hears his voice on NPR."

I click the off button. Fling the remote aside. Reach for the phone on the bedside table. But I realize I am in no mood to be put through a phone tree with NPR. Instead, I email the radio station, reminding the journalist that people died because of Russell Weller, that ten people were not so "lucky." I remind him that though this is temporary for some of us, others affected by impaired older drivers have lost their independence forever.

In a perverse way, Grotsky and the journalist give me permission to let loose my fury, to howl my grievances into the dank air, to shed weeks, months, of repressed indignation. Releasing all that anger feels much like recovering from a bout of food poisoning, and after sending the email to NPR, I fall back into the mattress, wrung out and limp, but a little less helpless.

Chapter 27

One of my doctors hands me a thirty-five-page photocopied text of the Book of Job. He asks if I've ever read it. Yes, I have. A lifetime ago. In Hebrew school, and when my father hauled us kids to temple on the High Holy Days. I raise an eyebrow at my doctor. *Why are you asking? And why now?*

"This is probably a good time to read it," he says.

Alone, back at Kathleen and Rick's, I examine each letter. B-o-o-k o-f J-o-b. It's been three months since the accident, and I haven't even thought about God's connection to it. But months later, for whatever reason, a haunting curiosity about God's role ruffles my sleep. From the bedside table, I dig out the copy my doctor gave me.

> The Lord said to Eli'phaz the Te'manite: My wrath is kindled against you and against your two friends; for you have not spoken of me what is right, as my servant Job has. Now therefore take seven bulls and seven rams, and go to my servant Job, and offer up for yourselves a burnt offering; and my servant Job shall pray for you ... So Eli'phaz the Te'manite and Bildad, the Shuhite and Zophar, the Na'amathite went and did what the Lord had told them; and the Lord accepted Job's prayer.

As I read the passage—five or fifteen times, then Google various interpretations—I finally decipher the meaning. Job's friends falsely claim his suffering is a consequence of committing grave sins. God is quick to reprimand them for their severe misrepresentation of His character. Despite their mistake, Job forgives his friends. God is happy with Job, and even extends His good graces to Job's friends. A startling notion dawns on me: maybe my doctor believes God is testing my ability to forgive. But it's hard to forgive someone you don't know, have never met, even if it is an old man who meant no harm.

Chapter 28

Though I question why I survived while others died, I don't ask God, "Why did Russell Weller drive into me?" While talking with a friend about the accident, the answer splashes over me like cold water. "Why not you?" she says. I give her a slow nod. I have to think about this. Was it meant to be that the ones struck were there at the right place and time? Were we all present that day as a result of our own free will? Was it meant to be that Russell Weller be the driver? Russell Weller the cue ball, the rest of us solids and stripes. And what role, if any, did God have in the crash? What were any of us supposed to get out of this? Some wonderful, fucking lesson from God? It's unbearable—the thought of God deliberately imposing such unmerciful acts on a human being. Simply to teach a lesson? Blood pounds in my throat, in my ears, behind my eyes.

Was it a lesson God couldn't wait to teach when a Dodge Challenger blasted through a crowd of counter protesters in Charlottesville, Virginia? Hundreds of far-right extremists invaded the city to protest the removal of a Confederate statue from a local park, making the public assembly the largest and most violent of its kind at the time. An avowed white supremacist, the driver, James Alex Fields Jr., carried out the cold-blooded attack, motivated by a deep-seated hatred for anyone he perceived as non-white. God's lesson? Or free will?

Why would God condone such a malicious atrocity, one that left thirty-two-year-old Heather Heyer dead and thirty-five others injured? I cannot bring myself to believe that God intended to teach a lesson when torch-bearing marchers assembled at the University of Virginia, spouting, "Jews will not replace us. White lives matter. Blood and soil." To think that God would use the Charlottesville attack as a teaching tool is ridiculous.

I can't imagine the other injured pedestrians in Santa Monica—or the families of Brandon, Cindy, Gloria, Diana, Lynne, Theresa, Kevin, Leroy, Molok, and Movsha—welcoming with open arms God's baffling lesson plan. Ten are dead. Lessons or tests of any kind will not bring them back. Ten also died in the 2018 Toronto vehicle-ramming attack. Lessons or tests will not bring back Beutis Renuka Amarasingha, Andrea Bradden, Geraldine Brady, So He Chung, Anne Marie D'Amico, Betty Forysth, Chul Min ("Eddie") Kang, Ji Hun Kim, Munir Abdo Habib al-Najjar, Dorothy Sewell. I can't imagine their loved ones are grateful for God's lessons. Who is doing the punishing? Who is choosing the lessons?

Chapter 29

I haven't even been living with Kathleen and Rick for a week when I twist around at the end of the bed, shift onto the commode, and hear, *plop.* It could not have come from me; I would have known. I lift myself with my arms and look down to see the source of the plop. My socks. My eyes bob from one side of the room to the other, desperate to find something in which to hide them. If I was able to run, I'd sprint like a cheetah from the shit-stained socks. That same morning, as Kathleen hurries toward the commode to empty it, I hold my hand up like a construction site guard. "Wait. My socks. They fell in."

"What? How did that happen?" Her face turns red. Is she angry?

"I'm sorry, I mean it. You know how cold it's been at night. I've been wearing my socks. But my feet, they got too hot. I kicked them off. They must have fallen in at some point. I don't know how it happened. Please, throw them out." I felt hot with humiliation.

"Stop it," Kathleen says. She shakes her head at me. "I'll wash them in hot water."

Later that day, I find the socks on my bed, folded with the rest of my laundered clothing, as white and terry-soft as the day I bought them. I slip them on. They're warm, as if they have just come out of the dryer. Kathleen not only wanted to wash my socks, she needed to wash them. As embarrassed as I am, I smile. *Shit happens.*

I stare into the full-length mirror. A thick-browed woman, with an anemic face and dark shadows under her eyes, stares back. I peer closely at her, trying to remember what she looked like before those shadows. I strip off my t-shirt and the purple yoga pants I've been wearing throughout the fall. Pushing against the wheelchair rails, I raise myself up off the seat. My upper torso stops at forty-five degrees. I push harder against the rails, forcing my spine upright. The muscles in my back and hips pull. I push again, this time stretching the muscles enough to stand straight. My arms shaking, I study the woman wearing baggy underpants. Her legs appear much longer than I remember, but her once sculpted quads now look like dowel rods. Her shoulder blades and hip bones resemble the nubby ends of chicken legs. Her collar and shinbones look as if they are about to puncture through her skin. *This can't be me.* But the wasted woman, with her sunken cheeks and hollow eyes, does not lie. *It is possible to be too thin.* I speak a promise to the woman staring back at me. "I'll eat more. I'll get stronger. I'll take care of myself."

"I didn't think you were supposed to do that yet," Kathleen says, as she walks into the room and catches me standing in front of the mirror. "It's only the middle of October." Startled, I drop back into the wheelchair. Since I'm progressing well, the orthopedic surgeon has reassured me that I'll be walking by the end of the month. "That means you'll probably be going home soon." Kathleen's voice quivers, tears dripping down her blushed cheeks into her mouth. I slouch lower in the wheelchair. She walks past me toward the living room, whisking aside the purple-flowered curtain, and slumps down into the rocking chair. Its joints creak. She gazes at the floor, the corners of her lips pulled down, her eyes then shifting focus toward the window facing the chickens pecking at the grass in the backyard. I wait for her to say something, anything.

"The kids are all grown up. Remember when you first met Ben. How old was he, eight or nine? Ainsley was twelve?"

I swallow her melancholy whole, fumbling for a response that will make her feel better. "They're still kids," I say. But what do I know? I don't have children of my own. Kathleen taps her fingernails on the arm of the chair, taps louder, faster. Is she angry? Insulted? Anxious? As I internally replay what I said, I realize she yearns to care for Ben and Ainsley—change their diapers, rock them, feed them—in ways they no longer need. Perhaps some of that empty space has been filled by my presence here. Kathleen fills up my water bottle every night, leaves clean towels and a basin filled with fresh water at my bedside every morning, and cleans the commode with Lysol every day. Because I can't reach my feet without pain rippling down my back and hips, Kathleen pumices my heels, washes between my toes, clips my brittle toenails, and, of course, bleaches my socks.

"It seems like yesterday when Ben and Ainsley were with me in my daycare," Kathleen continues. "Now, Ben's in fifth grade, and Ainsley will be in college in three years." She scrapes her fingernail into the wood of the rocking chair, as if she's digging for something.

—

The water up to my waist in the pool, I cling to the walker. "Stand on one foot then the other," the physical therapist instructs me. With one foot shaking against the bottom of the pool, and the other flapping the water, I wobble. "Now rock back and forth on both feet." My head feels woozy, and when I follow her directions to look up and ahead, I wobble again, steadying myself with slow, careful movements as I apply equal pressure to each foot. Gritting my teeth, I plant my eyes on the opposite side of the pool, breathing in and out, in and out, for the long walk forward. Fifteen feet. *Right foot, left foot,* the same mantra I spoke when hiking Mount Washington sixteen months ago. But now it takes several seconds before my feet understand what to do. Finally, my right foot rises a few inches off the concrete, but falls back down. Fine vibrations radiate through my toes, up my calf, into my knee. "Walk heel-to-toe," the therapist encourages. After ten steps, my arches cramp. I stop to flex them before continuing. More than halfway to the other side, my knees tremble. My face starts sweating. The therapist swims to me, cradles me in her arms and floats me to the edge, where I rest my head on cool tiles. Transparent blue swooshes against the walls of the pool. Leaning against a jet, heated water massages my belly.

A few days later, I climb five steps, from pool to patio. *Right foot, left foot. Right foot, Left foot.* Still wary of holding my head up, I watch each foot rise out of the water. Deliberately, I lift each leg. When my feet touch the ground, they no longer fall against the concrete, but land delicately, not even a splash. At the top of the stairs, walled in by steam and soggy towel smell, my body feels eerily light. No solid anchor. Goose bumps cover my arms and legs. I walk down the steps, planting each foot with intention. Back in the water, the goose bumps recede.

Less than one week after climbing out of the pool, I push the walker from the bedroom through the living room. I walk ten feet, wearing brand new sneakers.

Heel-to-toe.

Head up.

Eyes forward.

Beyond the commode.

Beyond the curtain.

Straight toward the window facing the Worcester Range.

I pause by the window before turning back. Mount Hunger appears much closer than on that day a few months ago, when I had to squint to see its peak. Now, I see myself hiking to the top, the leaves crunching beneath my feet, the streams trickling over rocks and between crevices. A history with a future.

I continue walking five, six times a day, despite Kathleen's earnest questioning. "I thought you were supposed to walk only three times a day?"

I don't just walk; I explore, navigate my surroundings like a constantly moving one-year-old, though with a walker. Tennis balls and all, I push my way past the purple curtain marking the entrance to my bedroom, through the living room and into the adjacent hallway, beyond the burbling fish tank, through the kitchen, stopping to sniff the melon on the counter, then out the back door to the driveway. Sometimes I stand next to my car, a navy-blue Subaru Outback, and wonder when I'll drive again—or if I'll have the courage to drive again.

Chapter 30

"Why don't you practice driving?" My friend Patty asks one afternoon. We're sitting on her back porch, talking about Thanksgiving recipes.

"I'm not sure I'm ready."

"It's almost November."

I don't believe I have enough strength to drive yet. But my goal is to return to the NICU after the New Year. I'll have to drive forty miles each way. For that to happen, I'll have to start driving sooner than later. At the same time, to even consider driving again, I have to suspend my belief that any car or driver can kill. I have to convince myself that all car crashes are rare, accidental occurrences.

"You're definitely ready," Patty says, and hands me her car key. *You've got this, Melissa. Nothing will go wrong.* My hand trembling, I take the key, and press it into my palm. The teeth are rounded and smooth, as if the key has taken on the shape of the ignition, like a new sneaker that eventually molds to a thirty-six-year-old foot. *Yes, I can do this.*

I practice shifting my right foot back and forth between the pedals before starting Patty's car. I feel like I am sixteen again, learning how to drive, but instead of Patty in the passenger seat, it is my eighty-eight-year-old grandfather, an easygoing, always smiling man with the patience of a yogi who, to my knowledge, had never been in a car accident, not even a parking lot scrape. I remember him showing me how to parallel park, how he slipped the car into a tight spot, not once bumping the curb or tapping the cars on either end, his eyes, his face, even the wisps of white hair on his earlobes seemed relaxed. When it was my turn to park, he sat quietly in the passenger seat, letting me take my time, which I did. I lined up the car with the one in front of us, cranked the wheel to the right, looked out the rear window, slowly backed up, backed up some more, bounced off the curb with the right rear tire, cranked the wheel to the left, pulled forward, backed up, hit the curb with the same tire, again pulled forward then backed up. The rear bumper was inches from kissing the car behind us before I came to a jarring stop, perspiring like a boxer just out of the ring. I looked at my grandfather.

"Great job," he said. "Keep practicing, and I know you'll pass your driver's test." I did keep practicing, and I did pass. But, right then, all I wanted to do was take a long, cool shower.

Sitting in Patty's car, I shift my foot back and forth some more.

"Take your time," Patty says. I push the gas pedal halfway, the brake all the way to the floor. Each time I press the brake, it moans. When I release it, it clicks. *Am I pressing too hard?* A distracting fusion of leather, rubber, and vinyl odors make my pulse beat erratically. It throbs in my throat. I roll down the window and take a deep inhale—musky-sweet leaf piles and fireplace wood.

With a little coaxing from Patty, I turn the key. Holding fast to the wheel in the ten-and-two position, I turn out of her driveway, then up the country road at fifteen miles an hour. No other cars. No one out for a walk. Pebbles crunch and twigs snap beneath the tires. My brain feels muddled, but my foot knows what to do. I stomp on the brake at the top of the steep hill and the car stops, the engine boiling down to a slow simmer.

I turn the car to face down the hill, but something beneath it creaks. I stop, and tap the brake a few times. No creak. As we descend the hill, I keep my foot lightly on the brake, pulsing it as the car picks up speed. This time pebbles fly and twigs pop, making me flinch. Back in Patty's driveway, the engine silent, I flop back against the seat, shaking out the cramps in my hands from gripping the steering wheel. Finger indentations linger in the leather padding.

Clapping, Patty bounces in her seat. "Now," she says, "why don't you drive back to Kathleen and Rick's house?"

Is she on acid? Driving on packed dirt roads is one thing, but a twelve-mile stretch dotted with wildlife crossing signs? She must be on drugs to think I can make it past the first wildlife crossing sign without having to pull over as my head goes crazy with images of the car colliding into Bullwinkle mad-dashing it across the road. (I've seen moose run, and they can run fast, believe me.) As I am about to twist the key out of the ignition and hand it over to Patty, a crow caws in a nearby maple tree. It caws again and again. I hear it telling me to stop being a jellyfish and drive already. Patty looks at me with a half-smile, and says nothing. Just to get away from the crow's pain-in-the-ass goading, I give in and start up the car with a snap of the key. Narrow winding roads, blind curves, school buses—and pedestrians. I stop several feet before a crosswalk, where a guard waves a stop sign. My toes pinch and my thighs twitch as I push the brake to the floor. In the center of Montpelier, I hunch close to the wheel, my eyes peeled for people leaping into the street. *Brake. Gas. Brake. Gas. Be ready to step on the brake.* A bicyclist, a jogger, a mother pushing a stroller, and a barking dog all compete for my attention. Again, I press hard on the brake to let pedestrians cross. *What if I miss it, and step on the gas instead?*

Three and a half months had passed since I had driven. I felt like a new, inexperienced driver. I couldn't seem to shake the fear of confusing the gas pedal for the brake. Part of my ongoing education about "pedal error" now included an unasked-for familiarity with everything associated with this term. I learned that pedal error can happen to anyone. However, it is far more likely to happen to people in two age groups: older drivers, or young and inexperienced drivers. It happened to a younger driver in Tulsa, Oklahoma, a sixteen-year-old with a learner's permit who hit the gas pedal instead of the brake, and crashed into an Arby's restaurant. It happened in Dallas. A teenage driver pulled into a parking lot of a Metro PCS store, turned left to park, accidentally hopped the curb, hurtled into the building, tore through a wall, and sent a customer and pregnant employee running from the oncoming truck.

In Kathleen and Rick's driveway, with the engine finally off, my thighs relaxed. I can feel my toes. I sink into the seat, the lumbar curve hugging my spine. Baxter runs up to the car, barking and wagging his tail. I open the door, rub his back, and let him lick my face. Even the normally unpleasant odor of wet dog doesn't stop me from accepting his congratulations for a successful first drive.

Chapter 31

Patty opens the front door, and I scoot on my butt across the threshold into the kitchen, then pull myself up, using the walker for leverage. I look around my apartment; no one has lived here for three months. I catch sight of the rectangular pewter case my father nailed to the doorpost soon after I had moved. Inside is a mezuzah, a tiny piece of parchment inscribed with prayers from the Torah. Both are reminders of Jewish identity and the oneness of God. I touch the Hebrew letters G-O-D etched in blue across the outside of the case, then withdraw my hand, as if I am pulling it away from a hot coal. But the letters are cold, as though they have not been touched in a long time. I can't remember the last time I touched them, or if I have ever touched them before today.

I stare at the letters, unsure of the reason for my vague feeling of fear and mistrust. I see my father hanging the case, his fist raised, banging the nails into the doorpost, the sound of his hammering startling me. POUND! "Remember, blood is thicker than water." POUND! "You can take time off work and come visit me more often." I back farther away from the doorpost. I take a long breath. My father believed the mezuzah is meant to protect my home, to keep me safe from evil spirits. I don't know what I believe, but I want peace from those images.

As I push my way into the kitchen, I smell dust and stale air—months of abandonment. A thin layer of dust covers the skier ornament dangling in the window, the cast iron pans hanging over the stove, the framed photos of antique gas tanks on the wall. The refrigerator hums. Alphabet magnets dot its door in disconnected phrases.

I step into the sparsely furnished living room: couch, recliner, coffee table, and boom box. No knickknacks, or heaps of magazines and newspapers. My apartment is lifeless, unlike my bedroom at Kathleen and Rick's, where friends and family left me with a library of celebrity enquirers, crossword puzzles, spiritual books, and self-help pamphlets. Where generous piles lay on top of the dresser, on the floor next to the bed, on the drop-leaf table at the front of the room. Symbols of love, empathy, and kindness.

Here in my apartment, the walls I painted sea green in June remain barren, and a hint of paint vapor lingers in the room. In the office off the living room, there are a second-hand area rug on the floor and three cacti on the plywood table by the window. The plants droop to their sides, their once pink flowers now wilted and brown. I pinch a clump of soil, and it crumbles between my fingers. "I'm so sorry," I say to the plants, wondering how someone could possibly kill a cactus. What should I expect?

As I shuffle back into the kitchen, I shield my eyes from the blast of sunlight. Squinting, I can see it. The calendar on the wall opposite the kitchen table. It still displays the month of July. On the sixteenth day, in my crisp handwriting, it reads, "Santa Monica." I blink a few times. Still "Santa Monica." Flashbacks to the morning before I left for the airport come cascading back: dawn stars sprinkling the eastern sky, the song of early robins, a five-mile run on dew-moistened trails. On the way to the airport, I stopped at the neighborhood gas station for my daily thermos of black coffee. "See you when I get back next week," I said to the owner.

Patty, who is watching my reaction, says, "Let's change the month to October." I lift the page, but pause at the photo of a field of strawberries gracing the top half of the calendar. I lean in closer, sniffing it, as if I can smell berries cooking in the sun. I flip three pages ahead to a photo of a walking path shadowed by crooked limbs of grand oaks crowned in melting gold. Just like that, time tips forward.

Quickly, I turn the pages back to the strawberries, compelled by the notion that it's possible to reverse time and start over again—for all seventy-three of us.

Chapter 32

On November 2, I call Kathleen at work to tell her I'll be moving back home. My neighbor down the street has offered to help with the move—three months of newly accumulated things. "Are you sure you're ready?" Kathleen asks. "I thought you said you'd be here until January." *I don't recall saying that. Maybe Kathleen's right. Maybe I'm not ready to go home.* But I have to return to my life; I have to get back to work as soon as possible. After a twelve-week waiting period, I started receiving long-term disability benefits through my employer in October. Though the monthly payments cover sixty percent of my regular salary, it isn't enough to cover all my bills, including the stockpiling of out-of-pocket medical costs. Within the first three months alone, the total cost of care, including charges covered by health insurance, amounted to nearly twice my annual salary.

I stare at the mishmash before me. Boxes of books, trash bags bulging with clothes, a paper bag filled with healing lotions and oils, a plant made of lollipops.

"Ready?" My neighbor startles me as she walks in and stands in the doorway to the room, her eager eyes taking inventory of stuff so easily accumulated, yet difficult to part with.

Still clasping the phone, I give her a thumbs-up. While she loads bag after bag into the truck of her car, I finish my conversation with Kathleen and reassure her that I'll call her later that day. I hang up, the heat from the phone lingering in my ear.

I stop for one last look before rolling out of the house. Everything—the blank walls, the bare floors, the naked mattress—take on a gray cast. Only the commode and Lysol stand out in contrasting shades of white and fluorescent yellow.

Unlike my tidy apartment I had visited a couple of weeks earlier, unpacked belongings now wait for me. The clutter feels daunting. In winter's dim light, frost tints the windows. Wind howls, driving cold air through the crack at the base of the front door. Treetop branches and twigs rattle the tin roof. My lack of mobility and fear of this old house catching fire convinces me to sleep on the pullout sofa in the living room, rather than in my bedroom on the third floor. A burn nurse never forgets children ruined by fire. Green eyes peering through charred faces. Blackened toes and fingers. Odor of burnt flesh.

I stay indoors much of that November, alone.

It feels as if my apartment is closing in on me; I need to get outside. It is Patty who temporarily rescues me from the clutter of boxes still to be unpacked. As we head up I-89 toward Burlington, to visit my coworkers in the NICU, bare trees wall the edge of the road, their limbs bending forward, kowtowing to the November wind. Snow carpets the upper ridges of Mount Mansfield and Camels Hump. Once again, the seasons have changed. For me, time has simply skipped ahead.

While Patty parks the car, I wait in the hospital lobby, watching weary visitors sprawled on couches or pacing the hallways. Healthcare personnel scuttle off to one trauma or another, their clogs clapping tile flooring. Code red announcements, crying children, and beeping pagers blend into a brew of sounds. As a hospital custodian passes, bucket in one hand, mop in the other, a sharp, eye-watering odor socks me straight in the face, routing me back in time to the Lysol Kathleen used to clean the commode. As emotionally potent as that scent is, a more alluring and reassuring thought washes over me. My visit to the NICU is the first step in getting back to work.

In the NICU, as I push the walker toward the front desk of the nurses' station, I smell construction paper, the smell of nostalgia. I look to my left at a corkboard tacked with baby photos, their faces pasted on light blue sheets of paper. I recognize some of the faces, the ones I had cared for, but others, I do not. Their faces have matured into those of toddlers. I brush my hand across the photos and stop at one with me and the plump face of a two-month-old, born at twenty-four weeks gestation. In the photo, I'm standing next to him in his crib, his head and back propped up by pillows. A basketball, twice the size of his head, balances on the mattress in front of his lap, so all you can see is his bald scalp and gray-green eyes. It's signed with the names of the NICU staff. I recall when I cared for him three years ago—a few weeks after he was born—and how, each time I would pick up all one-pound-eight-ounces of him and settle him against his mother's breast, it felt as if I were holding a small bag of confectionary sugar. I remember his fragility during those first weeks—his heart rate plummeting when changing his diaper, when repositioning him, when talking too loudly by his Isolette. I would feel a weakness in the center of my chest.

The preemie was discharged from the hospital sixteen weeks after he was born. As I stare at the photo of him, I recount the passage of time in my head. *Yes, he's three years old now, approaching four. He's walking, running.*

At the nurses' station, hardback, silver-bound charts lay scattered along the counters. Looking through the wide windows into the unit, I see that nothing has changed: Isolettes, prams, and beds with overhead heaters lined up in orderly rows. I feel grateful to be here, among my coworkers who have visited me at Kathleen and Rick's, brought me self-soothing goodies like foot creams, herbal teas, and candles, and donated their sick time after I had used up mine within the first couple of weeks of returning to Vermont.

A nurse looks up from a chart. Recognizing me right away, she gasps. A cluster of nurses sitting at the other side of the station startle. In unison, they jump up and gather around me, talking fast, asking how I've been feeling and when I plan to return to work. Hearing the commotion, another nurse walks out of the unit, holding a soiled diaper the size of a napkin. "I bet you don't miss this," she says. I laugh, and my mind goes back to the scent of adhesive tape, isopropyl alcohol, plastic IV bags. I remember the scent of Johnson-and-Johnson lotion—a newborn after her first bath. A distant cry distracts me. I stare steadily into the unit, wondering which baby needs attention. Marie, one of the nurses, asks, "Do you want to go in?"

"Really?" I want to go in; I don't want to go in. The cry grows louder, a please, come-pick-me-up cry. I step forward. The whoosh of a ventilator's mechanical breath and the steady ding of an IV pump summon me closer. I step over the threshold separating the nurses' station from the babies. Marie waves me away from the crying baby and toward an Isolette by the tall windows overlooking Burlington's Lake Champlain a couple of miles away. An orange light streams through the glass, creating a crisscross pattern of shifting shadows on the counter top. I look away from the dizzying shadows, out the window at the lake, which takes up much of the horizon. I turn back toward the Isolette, hover over it, and watch the sleeping preemie, wrapped like a gift in a pink-and-blue striped receiving blanket.

Blond wisps poke out from his narrow head, and a spaghetti-thin nasogastric tubing hang from his nostril. It doesn't seem to bother him. He keeps sleeping, sucking on the pacifier, the plastic ball on the end moving in and out, in and out. I had swaddled so many babies in receiving blankets, tucked their arms and legs in, as if stuffing a sausage, then inserted NG tubes into their doll-like noses and down into their stomachs. More often than not, they managed to unravel themselves, hook their tiny fingers around their NG tubes and pull them out. I didn't know then what it felt like to have one snaked into my nose, down the back of my throat, and into my stomach. I knew it had to hurt, because each baby always cried. But now, after having an NG tube while hospitalized, I know how much it hurts. I feel the razor blade sensation in the back of my throat and in the lining of my nose as I watch the preemie's tube slide in and out.

The memory of the cherry-cheeked face of a full-term baby I cared for more than a year ago rises in my mind. She spent many weeks in the same spot where the preemie I am now watching sleeps. Born with an omphalocele—an umbilical hernia—nearly all eleven feet of her intestines, along with her liver, stomach, and spleen, protruded through a three-inch opening in the center of her belly. On the night she was born, after I admitted her into the NICU, poked her heel for blood samples, poked her again to insert an IV into her scalp, the surgeons wheeled her to the operating room. They had hoped to tuck all four organs back into her abdominal cavity. But her organs were too swollen, and she returned to the NICU, her spleen and two-thirds of her intestines bulging from her belly, ten inches high. The protrusion was wrapped in white gauze and looked like a three-scoop ice cream cone.

Postoperatively, and for several days after that, she breathed with the assistance of a ventilator. A continuous morphine infusion kept her asleep during the initial few hours after surgery. But then she woke, her feet kicking, her arms wind-milling, her eyes scrunched shut, and her spine arched into a mini backbend. She made the expression of crying, her mouth forming a tiny O, but no sound came out; only air escaped from around the breathing tube. I injected an extra dose of morphine into the IV sticking out of her pink hand. Within seconds, she fell asleep, her limbs slack, her eyelids soft and still. A few hours after that, she woke again, her feet kicking, her spine arching into another backbend. I injected more morphine and notified the doctor on call. "We need to increase the infusion," I said. I adjusted it in micro-increments, listened for the slowing blips sounding from the cardiac monitor, and closely watched the see-saw movements of her chest ease, each breath like the hypnotic rise and fall of a wave on a calm day.

Eight weeks after she was born, she was discharged from the hospital. By the time she turned eight, she had undergone fifteen surgeries before her organs fit back inside her, before the hole in her belly closed for good.

—

I'm not sure I have it in me to care for babies again, if I'll be able to stop myself from feeling every bit of pain they feel. Is it even possible to divorce the memory of your own pain while trying to alleviate someone else's? If I can't separate an infant's pain from my own, I can't be the effective nurse I once was. Sometimes compassionate distance is stronger medicine than empathy.

My legs waver again. I grip the walker and sit down in the chair nearby, my legs still shaking.

The preemie in the Isolette starts squirming, and he opens his eyes. He stares at me. I stare back into his slate pupils reflecting crystal flecks of light. All dings, beeps, and cries seem to stop. The only noise I hear comes from him: a coo then a grunt. The pacifier falls out of his mouth and a wail reverberates off the walls of the Isolette. He kicks so hard the blankets unravel. Marie opens the porthole doors, and when she untapes his diaper, his wail is piercing.

As Patty and I head south toward Montpelier, I still hear the force of the preemie's cry in my head.

Chapter 33

My fractured foot still healing, I'm limping through the center of Montpelier with my ski poles when I see the thirty-something-year-old guy, the same guy I avoided two months ago while a friend was helping me with errands in town. I can't avoid him now—he's wheeling directly toward me in his chair. It will be too obvious if I turn the other way. Instead, I continue, thinking I can limp straight past him. But as we draw closer to one another, he stops, clicks the wheelchair brakes into the lock position and mumbles something to me. I can't understand what he is saying, so I don't respond. He tries again to vocalize what he wants to tell me, his neck tilting backward, forward, side to side, as he grunts out sounds that I still cannot understand. I step closer to him, and look down with my best pretend smile.

He brings his face close to the keyboard jutting out from the front of his wheelchair, and pokes at the keys with his contracted pointer fingers, his swollen knuckles cinder-red. The tips of his nails are round and smooth, as if they were recently trimmed. Noticing the spasticity of his movements, I am certain he did not manicure them.

I wonder how wheelchair users not only cope, but thrive, knowing they will never be able to walk, run, or hike. As an ignorant able-bodied person, I assume wheelchair users must be miserable. It is my therapist who sets my bent thinking straight. One day, long after the accident, as I'm walking into my therapist's office, his previous client is leaving. He is using a wheelchair. When I ask if he needs me to open the back door for him, he smiles and says, "Yes, please." He wheels forward, then backward, then forward again, inching the chair through the narrow hallway. I ask if he needs help. "It's all right," he says. "I got it." I hold the door open and wait until he rolls through. Just before he rolls down the ramp to the van that will take him back home, he nods again, smiling. "Thank you."

Remembering my own experience, I tell my therapist how sad I feel for his client.

"Why sad?" he asks.

"I don't know. I guess because it looked like he was struggling so much to get through the hallway. He has to face these kinds of barriers every day. How depressed he must feel."

"Melissa, here's something to think about. Maybe people using wheelchairs are a lot happier than you, maybe more than most of us walking too fast through life, rather than taking our time rolling along."

In Montpelier, the young guy pokes the keyboard again, this time causing it to bounce. I lean over his shoulder to read the typewriter font. "My name is Darren. What is your name?"

"Melissa." My voice trembles. "It's nice to meet you."

Darren pokes at the keys again. "Do you live around here?"

"Up the street. Right there." Hesitantly, I point toward the hill a few hundred yards behind us.

He swivels his neck around to see where I am pointing. When he turns to look at me, his head overshoots and seesaws back and forth.

He jabs at the keys again. "We should get together sometime."

"Sure," I lie.

I'm still afraid of his wheelchair. I can't bear to be reminded of my past limitations. I'm recovering in many ways—physically, mentally and emotionally—and in this circumstance, empathy requires a strength I am still not ready for.

I also lie to close the conversation, because Darren has to work so hard to communicate with me, and I don't know how to communicate back.

I step back, hinting that I need to get going. Darren waves, his hand flapping, as if it has its own, uncoordinated nervous system. But he doesn't seem to care, and beams with that same toothy grin I remember from before my days as a wheelchair user. I wave at him and limp away. I do not look back.

At what point along the peaks and valleys of the healing journey do you shed your victim mentality, your state of learned helplessness, a state in which you feel powerless to change your future? How do you trade that state of mind in for a productive one? For some, maybe staying mired in the familiar, even if it is nihilistic, is easier than stepping into the uncomfortably unknown.

I do not want to call myself a victim, and had made that clear in the letter I wrote to the Santa Monica Chamber of Commerce when I returned to Vermont: "I was a victim of the Santa Monica Farmers' Market tragedy.

But I am no longer a victim. I write this in order to share my strength with the other victims. They, too, will have long-lasting images."

I'm not sure the changeover from victim to survivor mentality has truly occurred for me. From observing his interaction with the world, I may have something to learn from Darren.

Chapter 34

"Hi Melissa. Hope all is well. I hope to go to McGillicuddy's on Thursday. Are you free?"

A whiskey-warm sensation fills my limbs. *Who is this guy, John?* Since the messages he sent in September, inviting me to play tunes with his band, followed by the open-ended, "lots to look forward to," he continued sending notes. "We're ready to have you play music with us. It'll be a good chance for you to get out and have some fun. If you need a ride let me know." I figure he's simply being a nice guy, nothing more. But he also has a knack for getting deep into my soul with his confidence and affirmation that, yes, I can play the fiddle again, that my existence reaches far beyond my injuries, beyond the fractured woman now limping along with a ski pole to keep her from falling. While considering getting together with him at McGillicuddy's two days from now, I realize I can't remember exactly what he looks like. The sultry June evening when I first met John seems so long ago, and yet I can still remember him eyeing me in my sundress as he sipped the foam from his Guinness, then licked his lips clean.

"Yes," I write back. "I'd love to meet up."

On the afternoon of our date, he calls. "How about dinner first, at Sarducci's?"

"Sure," I say. I'll meet you there." I need to drive myself. Really, with one belly-deep shout from my front door, you could probably order pizza to go. That's how close the restaurant is to my apartment. But it's December, and the ice, the four-foot snow banks flanking the driveway, and the poorly plowed streets make me second-guess my mobility. I stare at the phone, cracking my knuckles, wondering if I should call John back. What will he think of me if I tell him I'm afraid of driving down the hill, around the corner, less than a quarter mile? On a good day, I could send a paper airplane from my porch and land it square on the roof of Sarducci's. "Jesus Christ," I say out loud. "He'll think I'm a useless mess."

When I can't stand the indecision any longer, I pick up the phone and listen to the hollow dial tone for several seconds before pressing the keys. I poke the first three numbers, precisely and slowly, as if I am unlocking a secret code and need to get it right, then stop, motion to set the handset back in its cradle, stop again, take a deep breath and, finally, press the remaining numbers. The old-fashioned ring tone sounds once, twice, three times.

"Hello again." I pull the phone away from my ear, surprised by John's expectant voice.

I can hear him breathing, gently, like someone blowing on hot tea. I press the receiver tight to my ear. "Do you mind picking …"

"I'll pick you up at six-thirty."

I sink back into the couch, relieved. I have six hours to get ready, and read back through his emails, hoping I might learn more about him, why he has asked me on a date, a woman who has healed by leaps and bounds since the accident, yet has a lot more leaping and bounding ahead of her before she is fully put back together again. I stop at this email: "Funny, I have a burned image of you from the summertime when I met you many months ago. You were smart and had very deep eyes."

My heart dances a beat, more than a beat. I'm agog with excitement, eager to know what John meant by "deep eyes." No one has ever said that to me before. I want to know exactly what he saw in my eyes on that June night six months ago. Whenever I look in the mirror, I see glazed-over, constricted brown pupils, my lazy right eye wandering like a pinball.

The afternoon of our date, I shower, shave my legs, scrub my body with lavender bath gel, then slather it with lavender cream. An archived memory returns: The day a young surgeon walked into my room at LA General. I was shaving my legs. He blushed, his long eyelashes fluttering at me, and apologized for intruding. "I'll check in tomorrow," he said and turned to leave. "It's okay," I called out. "I'm done." I threw a blanket over my bare legs sticking out like oars from the hospital gown. He waved at me. "No, no," and reminded me again that he'd come back the following day. The next day came and went, but he didn't show up. A different, much older surgeon visited instead, and I missed the surgeon with the long eyelashes. I was hoping he'd see me as capable, vibrant, attractive, intelligent. I wanted him to want me. It is John's interest that reinforces that need for mutual want. His interest affirms that I *am* capable, vibrant, attractive, intelligent.

I rifle through the closet for an outfit, throwing aside baggy jeans and corduroys, tops that droop from my nearly non-existent shoulders, and a dress that hangs over me like a tent. A pair of olive-green slacks, the one pair that fits and doesn't slide down my narrow hips, will have to do, along with a matching top that reveals only a peek of my neckline. I comb my woolly eyebrows, brush blush onto my pale cheeks, hoping to cover up any sunspots, and thicken my eyelashes with brown mascara. Clumps form. I wash them off and start over. Looking at the made-up face in the mirror, the blush is too pink. I wash that off, brush on a lighter layer. I wait until the last minute to dab on earth-toned lipstick, but I can't refrain from licking the sticky stuff off my lips. What am I doing? Why do I have the makeup? I don't even know how to put it on, which is why I haven't worn makeup, unless ChapStick counts. I feel as if I am putting on a mask, trying to cover up something. I brush my hand along the left side of my forehead, where a purplish-black bruise once spread beneath my eye like an oil spill. But the bruise faded months ago. Even so, I can still see its shadow.

Precisely at 6:30, John arrives. As I open the door, I recognize him right away. The same wavy, salt-and-pepper hair and the stubble beard and mustache. Wearing jeans, a burnt-orange sweater, and a Donna Karan wool coat, he stands two steps below the threshold leading to my apartment, looking up at me through the doorway. "I'm short," he says. I like his silly humor, and hug him for it. The hug comes naturally to me. It seems to come naturally to him, too, because he hugs me back. I like his scent: Good & Plenty.

At dinner, the air around us is a marinade of olive oil, garlic, and grated Parmesan. Because we are sitting side-by-side, though, I can still smell Good & Plenty. "Are you still in physical therapy?" John asks, his eyes glimmering a hazel light. "Are you in any pain?" I keep my answers brief—"yes" and "not so much right now"—because I want to stay right here, with John, far from the accident, from the scars, from anything associated with Russell Weller.

As he lays his right hand on top of mine, his silver ring taps against my grandmother's gold wedding band. I gaze at the Celtic knot embedded in the ring. Trinity. The Father, the Son, and the Holy Spirit. It's covered with scratches, so I figure it's old. Maybe a previous girlfriend gave it to him. Or, since he has three daughters from a previous marriage, I wonder if the knot represents them. He catches me eyeballing the ring. "I've had this for years. I got it at an Irish shop in Burlington."

I nod, smiling, and sip some wine. Soon my head feels as if it's filled with helium, floating above me, away from me, toward some other, surreal place. I eat only bites of my salmon; John picks at his chicken Marsala. The food is incidental.

After dinner, we head to McGillicuddy's for a drink. As John reaches for my arm while I step out of the car parked in front of the pub, I look in the back seat, where I've thrown the ski poles I've relied on for the past month to keep me from tumbling onto the ice. The same poles that remind me of the winter before, and the three before that, when I skied four days a week at Sugarbush in Vermont, christening the morning with virgin tracks, planting the tips of my poles into packed powder, sometimes snow as fine as talc. With each parallel turn of my skis, I'd lift the poles into the brisk air, powdering my face white, and catch flakes on my tongue, tasting winter's breath mint.

"I don't need them." I look away from the poles, back at John.

"It's better than falling." He takes the poles and hands them to me. I poke them into the ground to brace myself, fracturing the ice into squiggly lines. I peer into them, dazed by the cracks, wanting to rupture the ice and bury the poles beneath the black concrete. "Are you okay?" John asks, looping his arm through mine. His closeness warms my brittle bones. He walks at my pace, our feet moving in sync, the ice shifting, making sounds as if it were singing.

We sit at the end of the bar, away from other customers. "What's your pleasure?" he asks, shifting closer to me.

"I'll have a Glenlivet. Straight up."

"Huh, a Scotch drinker." He flashes a smile so wide the gold crown protecting his molar flickers. He notices the miniature hurricane-shaped scar on my left hand, and tentatively touches it. "Is that from the accident?" His eyes mist. A shivering silence blows over us like a weather front. Then the Scotch comes. Eager to taste its bouquet, I take a sip. As it hits the back of my throat, I cough. It's been a good six months since my last dram of any kind of Scotch. I rotate the glass and take another sip, the familiar vanilla flavor lubricating my tongue and throat. For the rest of the evening, I forget about my miniature hurricane or any of my scars. I don't even think about my flaws.

Later that night, after our date, I check my email. "Peace for you Melissa. As pretty as the winter is, it felt like summer tonight. Who are you? My intuition says you're substantial. You'll surely make the world sweeter, and I hope and pray I catch some of it."

My heart tickles my sternum and ribs, each oxygen-rich beat blooming up the back of my neck, rewarming the memory of John's Good & Plenty scent. But I'm not sure what he means by substantial. Strong? I wonder if I'll be as strong as I was before the accident. And how does he know that I'll make the world sweeter?

Those self-doubting questions vanish when I read the rest of his message. "I'm free after 8 p.m. on the 24th, also the evening of Christmas, and the Friday after, maybe the Saturday after that. Just want you to know that I'm thinking about a plan to meet again."

We do meet again, on Christmas Eve. Between sips of wine, we sit on the couch in my living room, sharing our likes and dislikes, our fears and truths. "I'm afraid of flying and I can't stand the sight of blood," John says. "Oh, and I'm a Yankees fan and spend my Sunday afternoons at my parents' house watching football."

"I don't mind flying," I say, "and blood doesn't bother me one bit. Sorry, but I'm a Red Sox fan, and I could do without football."

We laugh.

When it comes to our deepest truths, John confides that he doesn't want more children. He's forty-six and has three older daughters, two who live with him three days a week, and one in college. He's ready to accept the next phase of his life.

Because he knows I'm only thirty-seven, and childless, he asks if I want kids. "No," I say, twirling the stem of my wine glass.

"Good answer. But I understand if you do."

"No," I repeat, this time a little more emphatically.

He doesn't ask me why I don't want children, as if he knows our second date is too soon for me to open up about that truth: that my mother left my siblings and me when we were young, and I had yet to resolve my anger and confusion over her leaving. And I don't want to have children, because I'm afraid I'll follow in her footsteps.

We share our bucket lists, too. John wants to travel to Ireland, to have a home with an outdoor fireplace, and to see his father turn eighty. The extravagant end of my list includes seeing a polar bear and swimming with a dolphin. First and foremost, I want to get back to caring for sick babies. But my goal of returning to the NICU by the New Year, less than a week from now, is not as reasonable as I had hoped. I still can't walk for more than fifteen minutes without experiencing the sensation of a dull nail shoved into my back, or a dart stabbing my left big toe. The lamp next to my side of the couch shines a candlelit orange, its incandescent warmth streaming toward us. With perfect intuition, John takes my hand in his, massages my fingers, their anemic nails pinkening under his touch.

Just before John leaves that evening, we are standing by the front door of my apartment when he leans down to kiss me on the cheek. As his lips brush my skin, I turn to face him. We kiss a long, this-is-going-to-work-out kiss. His lips are soft and taste like grapes. We stumble back from one another as if we are kids experiencing our first kiss. John's pupils dilate. I can see through them. I can see myself, my focused brown eyes, the right one that easily wanders now still and centered.

At twenty-three, I married a man who screamed at me if I made a mistake balancing the checkbook or folded the towels the "wrong way." I left him a year into our marriage. Yet, for the next several years, a hollow fear of loneliness trapped me in a cycle of relationships where I settled for being undervalued.

I didn't know then that bouncing from one dysfunctional relationship to the next was characteristic of "repetition compulsion," a Freudian concept describing how we unconsciously relive painful experiences from our childhood in our adult relationships. It's not that we are seeking painful situations; we are recreating the only world we've come to know. With daily support from family and friends, I finally found the strength to end a seven-year toxic relationship. My trip to California was how I planned to reward myself.

Unlike the others, John is interested in *me.* During our third date, he says, "I like to be needed. I need to be needed." I feel my skin loosen; my bones, tendons, and muscles soften under the warmth of his words. Given my circumstances—recovering from a physical trauma—being with John makes sense. I, too, need to be needed. I also need to be understood, and I sense that John hears me, sees me. All of me. Finally, I've gotten it right.

I know I've gotten it right when I read another one of John's emails. "I'm going to work hard to make sure we have fun and enjoy it and that you are safe and at peace all the while. I promise. Peace of the day."

I whisper "safe" and "at peace" into the candle-lit living room of my apartment. The S in "safe," the P and C in "peace" sweep across my lips, my tongue, my teeth. Since the accident, the meaning of safe has escaped me. Even years later, it still sometimes escapes me. Yet, John knows that's exactly what I need. To be safe.

Chapter 35

"Dessert?" the waiter at Sarducci's asks.

Too full, I decline.

"Let's take a look anyway," John says with a delicious wink, which I can't say no to.

"Okay, then. Why not?" Maybe the dessert list will be as enticing as John's wink. And we have reason to celebrate. It's March 18th, three months since our first date.

As I browse the menu, the items catch me by surprise. "That's strange," I say. "There's a Crème Melissa and a Melissa Tiramisu. And look at this, a Melissacotti."

Where is my head? Probably still floating in a cabernet mist from the one glass of wine I drank with dinner. If I was on the show, *Who Wants to Be a Millionaire*, I might use the Phone-a-Friend lifeline option to help me figure out why all the desserts are in my name. But I don't have to. With John right there, he is my lifeline. He points to the bottom of the menu. Printed in romantic font: "I will sing to you when you are young, will you read to me when we are old? Will you marry me my sweet, loving Melissa?" Bingo, I finally get it. This is not the menu.

That's when I hear live fiddle music in the background. I turn my head left, right, left again, toward the back of the restaurant. There's Katrina, John's band mate, slowly walking toward us, bowing a waltz, each note in perfect tune, the melody silencing all chatter and clinking of glasses and silverware. John lifts his hand up from under the table, holding a black velvet gift box. I slap my hand over my wide-open mouth, my oh-my-God-I-can't-believe-this-is-really-happening face. He hands me the box, and I cup it tight, shaking, stunned, stilled. It's warm, as if he has been holding onto it for a long time. Seconds pass, maybe an entire minute.

"Well?" he asks, "are you going to give me an answer?"

"Yes!" I yell. "Yes. Yes." Other customers, the waiter, the bartender, the kitchen staff, Katrina, all clap as if John and I have just played a hit song in a sold-out performance. I unclasp the lid. A round diamond, set in a platinum band, sparkles like a drop of spring water. John slips the ring onto my finger and rotates it side to side. Wearing the ring, I feel safer, as if nothing can go wrong. I gaze at the diamond. It transmits a light so intense that it reflects off my water glass, shining with yellows, pinks, and purples.

—

Five months later, on the morning of our wedding, heavy rains leave deep puddles along the pathway to the gazebo. "It'll pass," Katrina assures me. I believe it will pass, too, because John and I had chosen the 18th of August to be married, and the number eighteen in Judaism is *Chai*, meaning life—a representation of all the good things to come. We chose that day because our first date serendipitously fell on the 18th, the reason why John had planned our engagement for the 18th of March. Naivety aside, we chose the 18th to be married, because we believed it would shield us from future harm.

Moments before the ceremony starts, the rain miraculously stops. Sun-bordered, cauliflower clouds drift across the bluing sky. The ski poles that prevented me from falling six months ago are gone. I am strong, healthy, hopeful. Wearing a spaghetti-strap white gown, my head crowned in eighteen red rosebuds, and carrying eighteen long-stem roses cradled in my arms, I walk down the thirty-foot path, limp free. With his arm looped in mine, my father walks beside me, wearing a black tuxedo, his glazed-over stare fixed on the green lawn ahead of us. *What is he thinking? Is he worried?* My father's fingers curl up in mine, like the protective furl of a late summer leaf around a monarch. I believe my father knows John will always be there for me. John the summer leaf; me the monarch.

As my father and I walk forward toward the Gazebo where John is standing, the angle of sunlight spatters raindrops on the backs of chairs, creating a pearlescent glow. Heads turn and eyes well up. I glimpse Patty, as well as others who chauffeured me from one medical appointment to the next. Tina is missing. Work issues prevented her from traveling to the East Coast. Though I understand, I still can't imagine Tina not here, and envision her sitting in the middle row, wearing a white, scallop-sleeved blouse, the one I remember her wearing the day of the accident, but there's no trace of blood, no stains.

I slow my pace to smile at Kathleen wiping tears from her puffy eyes and blushed cheeks. The smells of rain, watered grass, and roses envelope me. The medley grows richer as my father and I approach the newly painted white gazebo, where John stands tall in his black tux, accented with a Venetian-red bowtie and cummerbund that match the roses. My father kisses me on the cheek and whispers, "I love you very much." He un-loops his arm from mine, and guides me toward John's extended hand.

Standing on the threshold of the gazebo, facing one another, John speaks his vows: "You will always have my trust and loyalty. I will be sure to listen to you. I will laugh with you. I will sing to you each day. I will always be on your side, always at your side."

Clouds drift past the gazebo, leaving a bright blue patch of sky above us. Bird wings whir in a nearby tree. I am standing in the center of an idyllic and comforting place.

"My dearest John," I begin. "As your forever Melissa, partner, and best friend, I thank you for waiting for my return, for giving me the best of days with promise of more to come, for being on my side, for listening to me, for making me feel safe."

In line with the Jewish tradition, John stomps on the cloth-wrapped glass, crushing it into fragments. All eighty guests clap, while my father shouts, "Mazel Tov!" and my mother waves at me as she dabs a dribble of mascara from the corner of her eye. I wave back, a tear free-falling down my cheek. John and I clink our goblets, sip wine—a burst of raisin. When John kneels to unwrap the cloth, I kneel with him, and touch a solid piece, fingering its beveled edge. Sturdy. A beginning, in happy contrast to the sliver of glass that emerged from my thigh nearly a year ago.

Part III

Chapter 36

Early in my recovery, my orthopedic surgeon said, "You'll be back in the NICU again." But fourteen months has passed since the accident, and the ice-pick pain in my back and hips persists. Walking down a thirty-foot path on my wedding day a month ago is one thing, but I can't imagine holding myself up for a twelve-, even an eight-hour shift. The dinging of heart monitors still lurks in my dreams. I wake every night at three in the morning, ready to feed a baby, and I long to hear and feel the familiar fabric of my career: a crying baby seeking my attention, a cotton receiving blanket against my arm as I hold a preemie, the diaphragm of a stethoscope between my fingers as I listen to the drumbeat of a newborn's heart. With every millimeter of a mother's breast milk I administered through her infant's nasogastric tube, I made a difference. I helped babies breathe easier when suctioning secretions from their endotracheal tubes. I relieved dying babies' pain when injecting narcotics. For fifteen years, assuming those kinds of duties defined me as a nurse. I can't imagine identifying myself with any other profession.

"You'll be a liaison to the district offices," a supervisor at the Vermont Department of Health says during my initial interview for a public health nurse position. "Your role will evolve and develop over time." Her ambiguous description puzzles me. I need to be needed. I need to find a way to re-claim my nurse status, regardless of the setting. More than that, because John's salary at the nonprofit where he works is not enough to pay all the bills, we need another source of income. To boot, it has been a year since I've started receiving disability benefits from my employer-sponsored plan, and a representative, who has not reached out once during that time, has recently called to question me on my progress. Why else would he call, other than to hunt for an answer that fits into the termination-of-payments checkbox?

During the second interview at the health department, the supervisor says I'll be writing protocols on maternal-child health issues, specifically on the care of chemically dependent mothers. I can't refuse. Plus, I'll no longer have to worry about babies surviving through the night, and because I'll be sitting at a desk, there will be little stress on my back. A few weeks after my first day as a liaison, my supervisor asks me to attend a meeting with other public health nurses at one of the district offices. I nod at her, as if I understand what my purpose will be at such a meeting, but I do not.

Driving the sixty miles to the district office, I'm on hypervigilant alert. The farthest I've driven since the accident: forty miles to Burlington to visit John before we were married. Even then, I drove below the speed limit, hugging the edge of the highway. Each time a car passed, I'd flinch and cling harder to the steering wheel. Before the accident, I drove that route three days a week to and from work, one hand on the wheel and a thermos of black coffee in the other, passing slower drivers at seventy-five miles an hour.

Now, as I head down I-89, sun rays beaming off the windshield, my eyes wide open, I focus ahead on the highway's broken white lines, maintaining the sixty-five-mile-an-hour speed limit. Each time a car engine revs as it approaches my blind spot, my body tenses and I dig my nails into the wheel. In my attempt to drown out the imagined sounds of cracking glass and metal against metal, I listen to Irish pub tunes. But my attention easily wanders to the repetitive hum of tires spinning against asphalt, and I see myself crashing through the windshield, lying on the side of the road, reaching out for help. I shift my attention to Killington's peak in the distance, where early-season saffron snow softens the drab browns and grays draping the steep-sided mountain, colors attributed to "Stick Season"—November in Vermont. But my mind is pulled back to the daunting reality that we have no control over how others drive. And we cannot always tell which drivers are sleepy, drunk, or inexperienced. Until it's too late.

Twenty miles into the trip, my eyelids twitch, and my head begins to bob to the side. I've become the sleepy driver. I roll down the window to let in the mountain air, slug down water from my Klean Kanteen, and munch on some almonds. Why am I so tired? Driving has never made me feel this exhausted before. Nearly a decade ago, while driving cross-country, I pushed on for hours, the window down so I could enjoy the wind caressing my hair and cooling my face. My eyes feasted on endless acres of farmland when driving through Iowa. As the horizon changed from yellow to orange, to red to purple, I wondered where all the land started, where it all ended. I was merely a speck in the midst of space. Driving used to be a way to experience beauty, a charge. Now it's a constant source of fear, an energy drain.

I've since become even more averse to driving, gladly letting John steer us around the bends and curves of highways on long road trips. Sometimes I close my eyes and nap, read a book, or work through a crossword puzzle, distracting myself from the frightening reality that I'm sitting inside a four-thousand-pound piece of steel machinery, and that there are trucks much heavier than our SUV that could flatten us in a New York minute. But John usually reminds me that being in a car, as a driver or passenger, is an opportunity to experience beauty. "Check out the purple sky," he might say. Or, "The daffodils are coming up over there. See those maples on the side of the road? The buds are popping."

The radiator in the room where the district meeting is held sputters a plume of steam every few minutes. My eyelids still twitching from the long drive, the heat makes me even more sleepy. I jot notes to keep myself awake. My brain is not able to shift into a high enough gear to make sense of seven other nurses discussing how the protocols they've been working on fit into the department's mission. I don't understand their vocabulary; it's far different from the NICU: no discussion about NG tubes, central lines, or anemia. Less than an hour into the meeting, my head feels as if it is filled with gel. I draw stars and moons and snowflakes, sketch random shapes and crosshatched lines. The nurses' voices sound distant, as if they are not in the room with me. Alone with the stars and moons and snowflakes, I draw more shapes: circles, rectangles, triangles. Anything to fill in the blank piece of paper before me.

On the drive home, I slide a CD into the stereo, hum "Brown Eyed Girl" and "The Star of the County Down." The electric-yellow lines on the highway start to appear as if they are wavering, like wind-blown ribbons, and flat light shimmers off the pavement, making it difficult to see far down the road. I turn off the radio, and morbid images appear at once in my head. *What if a deer or moose runs into the road and I don't see them? What if a moose crashes through the windshield? If I'm not killed, I'll suffocate.* It's too quiet, so quiet I think I could hear my brain chugging along as it tries to catch up with my runaway worries. Music has to help, so I turn the stereo back on and sing "Brown Eyed Girl" for fifty nail-biting miles.

Chapter 37

Six months later, my supervisor hands me my first review. The five-page document lists one compliment after another. "You have a broad view of the topic of chemically dependent mothers. Your work with the Sudden Infant Death Syndrome Project demonstrates your commitment to the health of children. Your clinical knowledge is a strong asset to the department." Even the director agrees. "Thanks for your good work," she scribbled on the last page.

But not long after that, a colleague scolds me for trying to push through a policy on the care of chemically dependent mothers too quickly. "This has been in the works for years," she says. "You can't expect to have it approved today, or next week." I hold the phone away from my ear, thinking she must be talking to the wrong person. I hang up, still not sure what she meant. I glance at the papers piled on the corner of my desk, turn away from them, glimpse the stack on the floor: changes in the hierarchy of the health department I have yet to read. I snap up a piece of paper from my desk, crumple it into a tight ball, and slam-dunk it into the hard-plastic trashcan by my feet.

My supervisor meets with me to discuss the apparent confusion. "It would be a good idea if you write protocols on basic, maternal-child health issues," she says. "Don't worry about the one for chemically dependent mothers." Nine textbooks are stacked on my desk. I thumb through them, reading the latest recommendations on postnatal care for mothers and their newborns. One book recommends one thing, another something else. I type an entire section of a protocol one day, delete it the next, type a new draft, delete that one, start over again. "How's it going with the protocol?" my supervisor asks two weeks after our meeting. "I have another one for you." My mind fizzes with rising fear. *What happened between the positive review and now? Have I lost my confidence, or is something wrong with me and I've just been covering it up?* When she walks away, I lay my head on the mess of papers spread across the desk. For the next several weeks and months, I feel as if I can't catch up.

Nearly a year after my first day at the health department, my supervisor informs me that as part of my public health role, I am to begin my orientation at the local clinic for Women, Infants, and Children. On the morning of day one, I sit in a hard folding-chair for two hours, watching a nurse interview a teenage mother while filling out a multipage form to determine her eligibility for WIC. She asks for her income, if she has any medical issues or nutritional needs, and if she is receiving any federal or state assistance. The mother rattles off numbers and names as she pops a bottle in her newborn's mouth, trying to quiet his cries. He spits it out onto her lap and cries louder. The mother picks up the bottle and drops it into the stroller. "Shush now," she says, "shush," bouncing her legs, her son jiggling up and down like a bobblehead toy. She tries patting his back before plugging his mouth with a pacifier. It falls out. He cries louder, not the kind of cry begging for a diaper change or to be fed, but an irritable, my-stomach-hurts cry.

Part of me wants to reach out for him, hold him until he stops, because that's what nurses are trained to do. But a greater part of me wants to run away from the inconsolable baby, the windowless room, the xenon overhead lighting, the bongo drumming in my sinuses. But how is the WIC clinic any different than the NICU? Though at times I wanted to run away from the NICU, I worked for twelve, sometimes sixteen hours at a time, indifferent to the noise and bright lights. I could easily do things like start an IV or change a dressing, and not flinch at the cries of other babies. Sometimes so many cried at once, I couldn't tell which one was my patient. Despite the commotion, I managed to listen to babies' skipping heart beats through a stethoscope, listen to their lungs crackle and wheeze, write detailed progress notes, explain procedures to parents, speak to parents on the phone, and hear every word they had to say.

That afternoon in the clinic, I sit in the same hard chair for another two hours, listening to another teenage mother report to the nurse that she lives with her nineteen-year-old boyfriend who works part time at a fast-food restaurant. He barely makes enough money to feed himself. The nurse asks her if he drinks the milk and eats the cheese the clinic has given her. The teenager sighs and rolls her eyes at the nurse. "No," she says, looking up at the ceiling. I wonder how I'd handle this situation. Would I nudge the teenager to tell the truth? Or pretend I believed her? But by that time, I am ready to get out of here, to lay my soggy head on a cool pillow. When I leave the eight-hour shift, my eyelids droop, as if someone were pressing down on them. I feel as if I haven't slept in two days. My hamstrings and hips are tight; all of me is tight, like I have been stuffed into a box for eight hours, then pried out and expected to stand up straight again.

Because I continue to experience physical symptoms—back pain, hip pain, foot pain—from my injuries, my gait is off balance, and I still see a physical therapist periodically for what I call a "tune up."

During the fourteen months I've been away from the bedside as a nurse, something about me has changed. The psychologist who visited me after I returned from California to Vermont explained that the nightmares and my hypervigilant state—fear of driving, fear of fire, fear of coming down with a fatal illness—are all symptoms of PTSD. But my brain's gas tank quickly empties each day. Is it fatigue, or do I no longer trust myself as a nurse? I know there must be more than PTSD to blame for my "rewired" brain.

I return to the WIC clinic the following day, thinking I need a little more time to re-acclimate to the xenon lighting and shrieking babies. But the lights make me dizzy, and when the nurse I shadow sticks an infant's toe with a lancet, his shrill cries echo off the low ceilings, into the cold examination room, into my ready-to-explode brain. It's as if someone is sticking needles in my ears. I still hear infants wailing long after my shift in the WIC clinic has ended.

"I can't go back to the clinic," I tell my supervisor the next day.

She agrees. "I think you'll be more productive in the office working on specific projects."

But she asks for medical documentation stating exactly why I can't return to the clinic. After much prodding from my psychologist a few months ago, I started seeing a PTSD specialist. She writes a letter excusing me from clinic duty.

> Ms. Cronin was in an automobile accident that resulted in severe physical injuries and PTSD. Symptoms of this illness include moderate to severe anxiety when overstressed and cognitive challenges such as difficulty concentrating and poor memory. When asked to assume duties in the WIC clinic, she felt overwhelmed with anxiety and dread. She also experiences anxiety when driving long distances, which triggers memories of the accident. As PTSD is a chronic condition, I'm unable to give a time frame when she can be expected to perform added duties.

The therapist discussed the effects of PTSD with me, but this is the first time I see them written down, in indelible ink. I've been turned inside out. Shaking the letter, as if I can shake off her words, I want to tear it up, shred it, never let my supervisor read the words "PTSD is a chronic condition." I pull at an edge, anticipating the crisp tear of satisfaction. Then stop.

My aunt visited me at Cedars a few weeks after the accident. She told me she had recently moved to the desert outside of Los Angeles, because the sounds of plane engines sent her into a panic, dragging her back to September 11, 2001. Through dust and debris, she scrambled her way down eighty flights of the North Tower. At the time she visited me, I didn't understand that her brain had been rewired to be on alert for every sound, sight, and smell that reminded her of that blackened day. I didn't understand why she sat on the edge of her chair by my hospital bed, ready to leap up at a moment's notice, or why she rarely blinked, as if doing so meant missing an urgent detail alerting her to run. Once, when she wheeled me into an elevator and the door closed, she yelled, "I think I smell smoke. We need to get out, now." She stood in the corner, her hands braced against the walls, her eyes shifting from me to the floor, to the ceiling to the doors. "What are you talking about?" I asked her. "I don't smell anything."

I do not tear up the therapist's letter. I know my PTSD symptoms are real. The night sweats, the gasps and screams when startled by anything: a yelping dog, a blasting siren or beeping horn, a ringing telephone or a bright autumn leaf floating past my line of vision. Hypervigilant, I watch for runaway cars. I even smell smoke when there is no smoke.

Chapter 38

The PTSD therapist I started seeing is the only one I know in Vermont well-trained in EMDR, or Eye Movement Desensitization Reprocessing. The treatment was originally designed for individuals with mental health conditions resulting from a traumatic experience. During the treatment, the client focuses in small doses on both an emotionally disturbing event and external stimulus at the same time. Therapist-directed lateral eye movements are commonly used as the stimulus, but other stimuli also work, like hand tapping or audio stimulation. The idea behind EMDR is to facilitate the accessing of traumatic memories, bringing that information to the forefront, along with newly-formed memories or information. The new, more positive associations forged are thought to help clients become less disturbed by the negative thoughts and images. These new associations also help develop cognitive insights. Theoretically, treatment is usually completed in eight visits, but the number of sessions needed depends on the client's history.

It's a spring day in 2005, nearly two years since the accident, when I walk into my first appointment, imagining a magically changed Melissa. A Melissa with an even heartbeat, steady breath, and calm body. But I fear that I will leave the appointment the same traumatized Melissa. A Melissa with a fluttering heartbeat, shallow breath, and hyper-startle even in response to a good-morning-I'm-off-to-work kiss on the cheek from John. The therapist warns me of the potential risks of EMDR: heightened memories of the trauma, and intense emotional and physical sensations. When I share with her my history—the loss of a mother figure at a young age, childhood abuse, a near drowning incident at fifteen, a skiing accident in my early thirties, emotional abuse by intimate partners, witnessing patient trauma and death—she explains that I likely have complex PTSD, which is typically seen in prisoners of war, concentration camp survivors, survivors of chronic abuse, or anyone who has been subjected to totalitarian control over prolonged periods. Again, I cannot deny or hide from what is real. My symptoms of complex PTSD tell the story: amnesia of both the Farmers' Market accident and my father's chronic abuse, reliving traumatic experiences through intrusive thoughts and nightmares, guilt over why I survived the accident while others died, self-blame for my failed relationships and my mother's leaving.

With a diagnosis of "complex" PTSD, the therapist explains that it can take several treatments before I see improvement in symptoms. Definition of "several treatments": one year of twice-monthly sessions.

During the first session, I sit back in a La-Z-Boy, feet up, with TheraTappers—transistor-like radio devices—tucked beneath the backs of my thighs. I hold the handles attached by wires to the TheraTappers, and over three minutes, at regular intervals, fine vibrations alternate beneath each hand. "If you feel anxious at any time," the therapist reminds me, "remember your safe place." *Calm water. Suspended in a warm bath.* While sensing the vibrations, I try focusing on the details of the crash. But my memory of the accident itself is empty, like a hollowed-out pumpkin.

I recall my last memory—the peach in my hand. As the therapist instructs, I close my eyes and imagine the rest. Screams. Flickers of something like heat lightning. The Buick charging toward me. Steel poles smacking against the ground. The taste of blood even though there is none. Impenetrable blackness. *Pop.* My body flying forward. I hit the pavement. Gravel and glass scrape and cut into my legs and arms. Something snaps. My back? I'm curled up on the hot asphalt. Then I reach for the cuff of Tina's sleeve. "Please don't let me die." But it was Tina who told me I had spoken those words. It was Tina who said that she found me lying on the pavement, reaching out for her. And it was Tina who told me about the poles smacking against the ground, about the screams, the racing Buick.

I have experienced a kind of memory conformity, when an individual's sharing of a memory influences another's recollection of the same experience. By internalizing Tina's memory, I make it my own, believe I have actually remembered the chaos unfolding around me when, in reality, Tina is the one who instilled into my gray matter many of the chilling details.

Those three minutes of EMDR feel like twenty before the therapist turns off the tappers. I share the images of me on the ground and the physical symptoms I experienced during the session: shortness of breath and a fist-tight stomach and chest.

"Now try to replace those thoughts with positive ones," she says.

I'm alive.

I survived.

I'm okay.

Another three minutes. This time the vibrations run deep into my fingers and hands. I picture myself soaking in a bathtub filled with warm water. My legs rise from the bottom, float, unencumbered. Lavender beads exfoliate old skin between my toes, the room itself filling with steamed lavender, unclogging my sinuses. I rub my hands along my arms, slide them over my belly, down my legs, feel the satin finish of my skin.

Foggy-brained by the end of a few sets of EMDR, I'm unable to articulate an exact emotion, but when I exit my imaginary bath, my skin feels taut, as if I might split apart. As I walk out the therapist's back door into the damp air and the odor of horse manure, my stomach and chest are still tight, but not fist-tight.

Waiting for John to pick me up, I approach the therapist's barn, where a horse sticks his head through the stall window. He snorts as I step closer. I hold my hand under his wet snout for him to sniff. He laps my palm with his beefy tongue, laps it again, harder, as if he wants to absorb every ounce of my anxiety.

Chapter 39

A few days after submitting the EMDR specialist's letter to my supervisor, I pass the conference room, its door ajar, and hear the department's director speaking my name. I stop, pretend I'm filing paperwork in the cabinet nearby. "Melissa needs to be fired," she says. I almost drop the fat file I'm fumbling with onto the floor. No employer has threatened to fire me before.

"Wait," I hear my supervisor say to the director. "She's a good fit for research projects. I think you should reconsider."

I tremble. The room turns blurry. Unsteady, I walk back to my desk, my head down, clutching the files. I fall into the chair and shuffle papers from one pile to another without reason. Other nurses walk past my cubicle, their high heels squeaking against the carpet, their blank faces looking straight ahead. Phones ring. Paper jams in the printer nearby. I stare at a protocol I've been drafting, but the flow chart of circles and squares and arrows make no sense to me—hieroglyphic shapes and symbols. My hands shaking, papers float from them, fanning out along the carpet..

I pick up the phone to call John. "Are you sure she was talking about you?" he asks.

For two weeks, I sleep only a few hours each night, but continue to go to work. John and I need the money. Between reading policies and drafting a protocol for SIDS (Sudden Infant Death Syndrome), I shuffle paperwork from one pile to another. I hide from the director, stay away from the copier near her office, and choose the long way from my cubicle when walking to my supervisor's office. I sit in the back of the room during department meetings, or miss meetings altogether. But after two weeks of little sleep, of coworkers asking why I've been unusually quiet, why I've missed meetings, I can't hold back any longer. With a sense of urgency so powerful, I feel as if I'm a revving engine, and finally tell the director I need to speak with her. "Sure, have a seat," she says, sitting behind her rosewood desk wearing a full smile. I drop into the chair, facing her from the other side of her desk, and confess what I heard her say behind the door. Her smile goes flat. She clasps her hands together on the desk. "You're not fulfilling your job description."

I'm not sure what she means. My job still seems to be evolving, though I don't know in which direction. My direct supervisor wants me to write maternal-child health protocols. The director wants me to work in the WIC clinic.

"When I get over-stimulated, it's hard to concentrate." I clench my hands beaded in sweat. "I get tired and easily confused."

"You'll be evaluated in three months," she says. "If things don't change, the firing process will take place."

Silent, she stares at me with narrow eyes. I glower at the 8 x 10 award in its grapevine wood frame and anti-glare glass, hanging on the wall above her, acknowledging her contributions to public health over the past couple of decades. I walk out of her office, the image of her award enlarged in my head, wondering if she considers PTSD to be a public health concern, a real diagnosis, or something contrived.

I begin to wonder if I actually have PTSD; maybe I've been making it up all along. Maybe the EMDR specialist is wrong. After all, coworkers say, "You don't even look like you were hit by a car."

Chapter 40

No, it does not look like I've been hit by a car, but the Buick still accelerates, again and again, through my mind, where others cannot hear the screams or see the damage left behind in the wake of the crash. Others cannot feel the aftershocks that disguise themselves as health crises.

Six months after the accident, when visiting my father in Florida, I still fatigue easily. All I want to do is lounge under a palm tree, read a long book, sip on iced tea. But he wants to do things with me. "Let's go to the market at Delray Beach," he suggests. He means the outdoor market.

I remember my visit with Kathleen and Rick to the Montpelier Farmers' Market five months earlier. I couldn't see the zucchini and kale, only the cars facing the market's entrance. I insisted we leave.

"Dad, I'm not up for it."

"Come on. You'll love all the crafts, and the food." I want to ask why he can't understand my reluctance, but I know he won't. I don't feel like explaining to him what I do not yet fully understand myself: PTSD.

At the Delray market, people push past me, elbows poking my ribs, full shopping bags jostling me aside, carriage wheels bumping my heels. The sun, huge and bright, makes me keep my sunglasses on. Still, my eyes ache. My stomach hurts. It's been four hours since I had breakfast: a sixteen-ounce cup of black coffee with two Sudafed for the head cold that won't quit.

I scan my surroundings like one searching for the closest fire exit in a movie theatre. I turn. My eyes settle on the far end of the street, on the plastic sawhorses, the only barriers in place to stop out-of-control cars.

"Why are you walking so fast?" my father asks as I hurry into a tent of watercolor paintings. As if doing so would protect me from cars. A large painting, saturated with swirls of reds, greens, and purples, makes me light-headed. The painting looks wet in the humidity, the colors about to ooze down the canvas like Dali's melting clocks. I step back, but the smell of acrylic polymers follows. I have to sit down, soon. "Dad, I think we need to leave."

"Maybe you need some lunch." He suggests an Italian restaurant two blocks away.

As we push through the crowd, I try to control my breathing, but the air is suffocating. We leave the market and stop at a bridge overlooking an inlet. I lean over the railing, enjoying the breeze blowing aside stray hairs from my forehead. I let the salt mist coat my face as I sway back and forth in time with the ebb and flow of jade-green waters. The ocean sounds as if it is whispering. "Hush, hush, hush."

At the restaurant, people keep bumping into my chair. A waitress passes us with a tray of meatballs that smell burnt. I can't catch my breath, and my heart is pumping hard. I dip a piece of bread in some olive oil and garlic, thinking my father is right—all I need is food—but the bread catches in my throat and I have to cough hard to get it out. "We need to leave, now. I don't feel right."

On the way back to my father's place, we hit every red light, and at one point get stuck behind a car bouncing to the beat of blaring rap. I check my pulse. *One hundred? One hundred-twenty?* Too fast to count.

"Dad, I think I'm having a heart attack. Maybe we should go to the hospital."

"Are you sure?"

I stiffen, grope for the car seat.

"Okay. Whatever you want." Staring ahead, my father tightens his hold on the wheel, turns right, away from traffic, toward Delray Medical Center.

"How far is it?" I ask. "How long will it take to get there?"

"Melissa, I'm going as fast as I can."

More red traffic lights. Ten seconds of red. Twenty, thirty. *Hurry up. Change.*

As my father pulls into the hospital parking lot, my heart rate moderates to a countable beat, and my breath slows enough so that it can now pass through my upper airway and into my lungs.

"Dad, maybe we should wait a few minutes before I go in."

"Like I said, whatever you want to do."

This acquiescent response from my father is new to me, so I'm not sure how to interpret it. But how can he say no to his freaked-out daughter? He has never seen me in the throes of panic before—I've never experienced panic to this extreme—so he has no reference for how to respond. Instead, he's just frightened enough to default to being supportive, which serves him well.

Mandeville flowers line the outside of Delray Medical Center's emergency room entrance. Fat, deep purple petals bow in the exhaust left behind by cars pulling up to the curb. My heart starts beating hard again, as if it's a fist punching through a wall. I want to tear apart my skin, peel it open, run away from myself. My breath grows rapid and my fingernails turn the same color as the flowers.

"Dad, do you think I should go in?"

"I don't know what to tell you."

This time his non-answer is of no help.

I can't convince myself that I'm at almost no risk for heart disease: a nonsmoking thirty-seven-year-old who pedals on a recumbent bike four days a week, swallows a fist full of vitamins every morning, eats salmon three days a week and leafy green vegetables every single day. What I am experiencing feels exactly like what I know to be a heart attack.

"Okay, let's go in," I say, and fling open the car door. My father trailing behind, I rush toward the entrance, push open the heavy glass door, away from car exhaust, into the sterile air.

In the waiting room, older people with smoke-white hair and dowagers' humps sit in orange chairs the shade of prison jumpsuits. I wonder how many of them drove themselves to the ER. An ashen-faced man sits across from us, holding his wife's hand. The skin below his sunken eyes looks like parchment paper, and the flesh around his arms hangs loose, as if he is wearing a shirt a couple sizes too large. He stares ahead at nothing in particular. How long has he been waiting? Why did he come to the ER? The flu? Pneumonia? A stomach virus? I know what these kinds of illnesses can mean for someone his age.

Within minutes, my fingernails change from purple to pink. My father waves at a nurse passing us, tells her that I am a nurse and I need to be seen as soon as possible. He is doing what I need him to do as a father—helping me in a way that shows he understands my fear. Still, I drop my head in my hands, utterly embarrassed by my father calling attention to himself and to me. Because I have yet to kick his past abuses and indifferences out of my mind's bedroom, my childhood bedroom where I once cowered under my father's metallic rage, all I can think is that I've inconvenienced him. *He probably wants to get out of here.*

The nurse guides me to a triage room, where she takes my blood pressure and heart rate. The red numbers on the automatic pump blip for a long time before stopping at 118/66 and 79. Average. Healthy. Or, as health professionals say, "Within normal limits." I feel anything but normal.

After leaving the ER, I call my doctor in Vermont. She phones in a prescription to a local pharmacy for Xanax. That same night, I lie in bed, rolling the minuscule white pill between my fingers, wondering if I should take it. *I'll take half. A quarter.* The longer I play with the Xanax, the longer I look at it, the more I imagine the power the tiny pill possesses. *It might put me to sleep for good. I might wake up confused, lost.* I know those thoughts are downright ludicrous. Really, for a nurse who has administered similar medications to babies and has witnessed them wake in the morning, the same babies, with the same dimples, the same coos, the same smells of breast milk on their breath. I need to get some sleep, and I place half a pill on the front of my tongue, hold it there for several seconds, its chalky coating dissolving into my taste buds. I curl back the tip of my tongue, drag the pill into my throat. Swallow. I sleep the entire night, dreamless.

The panic attacks continue. In the thick of them, I don't associate the symptoms with panic but rather as a reaction to something I've eaten. The December after John and I are married, while my mother is visiting, and she and I go out to dinner, we share a slice of chocolate cake for dessert. It tastes like dark roasted coffee. After a few bites, the hotspot lights up, flares like a sparkler. I try to think of something else, like what movie we should rent that night, a comedy or a drama. By the time we get home, my body shakes uncontrollably. Lava fills my throat. I think I'm choking. I've never experienced an allergic reaction to chocolate before, but I believe I am now. When I stand up, I feel the floor shift and latch onto the back of a chair. I recite what has become my standard call for help when convinced that I am dying. "Mom, I don't feel right. Something's wrong." I stumble to the phone across the room and dial 911.

She jumps up from the couch like one of those jack-in-the-box toys, her arms and hands open, as if she is begging to be told what to do. I crouch by the front door and wait for the rescue workers to arrive. My mother runs to the door and stands over me, her gaze darting from me to the door, then back to me.

"Are you okay?" she asks. "What do you want me to do? Tell me and I'll do it."

"I need to call John."

She wants so much to help. And how much I want to give her that maternal moment. But I don't trust she'll know what I need.

It is John's enduring presence I trust. The day before our wedding, I had a panic attack after eating a few bites of crab salad. Convinced it was due to an allergy to shellfish, I asked the server at the restaurant if they had Benadryl, to which she said no. Again, I thought I might die. My mother, who was with me at the time, offered water and more food: "You haven't eaten much today." But I insisted we go back to the inn where the wedding would be held, and where I had conveniently left the Xanax. I called John. "I'll be there in less than twenty-four hours, my lovely Melissa." He stayed on the phone with me for thirty minutes, even though he had to pack for the wedding the next day, pick up wine for the reception, and follow up with his friends who would be performing music at the ceremony. When I had a panic attack during our honeymoon, John sat with me in the hotel room until I slept off the exhaustive fallout of the panic and the sedative effects of the Xanax, which he had to convince me to take.

Though the ambulance station is less than two miles from our house, it seems to take too long to arrive, and my mother starts pacing. I stare at my watch, the second hand slowing down between the twelve and the three, slowing again between the three and the six. I press my finger into my wrist pulse. Blood pounds against my skin. I see the vessel pulsating. Minutes after four EMTs arrive, I hear John's heavy steps in the hallway. He dashes through the open front door towards me sitting on the couch, and takes my hand. The heat in my throat cools; John's touch shoos away the rabid animal inside me. One of the EMTs checks my pulse. "Perfectly normal," he says. "It looks like you had a panic attack." I turn away from the EMT and look at John. "I'm sorry."

"It's fine. As long as you know you're okay." He pulls me close to him. I turn my face into the warm center of his solid chest, into the echo of his vow he made on our wedding day. *I will always be by your side.*

That night, again with John's persistent encouragement, I take a Xanax, just in case. I sleep all night, with him beside me, the smooth sole of his foot against my calf.

—

At least EMDR gives me the self-soothing techniques to cope. When I become consumed by irrational thoughts, when I lie awake at night thinking John is dead because I can't see his chest rising and falling in the dark, I'll do as the EMDR specialist encouraged. I'll say, "STOP." And the hidden hand strangling my esophagus will release its hold. EMDR has also helped me control some of the nightmares. Each time my voice strains against the pressure in my chest, I think my way out of the typhoon-like swirl. *This is not real. This is not real.* And when I wake in a cold sweat, panting, I say out loud, "This is not real. This is not real."

Still, for years, I carry Xanax with me wherever I go: to the grocery store, on road trips, when flying. Simply having it with me is a remedy. In the pouch of my backpack, in the side pocket of my fleece, in my oversized wallet, the Xanax provides comfort. All I have to do is look at the amber bottle, shake it, hear the pills jingle against the plastic walls. Occasionally, I twist off the cap to be certain they are still there, then pour the pills into my palm, and count them, twice. Fourteen minuscule white pills, the shape of life rafts, rafts that rescue me from heart attacks, allergic reactions, and infections. The only time they are not with me is during my recurrent nightmares: *A car launches into the air, then crashes to the ground. It rolls onto its side, glass shattering. It rolls again, toward me. I run, faster, faster. . .*

Chapter 41

Sitting at the kitchen table in John's apartment, I filled myself up with spoonful after spoonful of butternut squash soup seasoned with rosemary and Granny Smith apples.

"Wow, John, you made this?"

"Yes, I did."

"I had no idea you were a cook."

"I take after my mother."

Eating that soup was a baptism of sorts. A couple of months had passed since our first date, and it was the first time I tasted food John had labored over for me. He had peeled and sliced each apple, peeled and chopped the squash, stirred the soup thick, mingling the flavors like a party host introducing compatible guests.

"John's love soup" I called it.

Now, six months into our marriage, and living in our new condo, he has quickly assumed the role of cook in the family, following his mother's Ukrainian recipes: poppy seed bread, pierogi, halupki. He inherited all kinds of international cuisine from his mother, including Mexican, Puerto Rican, Italian, and Cuban.

On Saturdays, John wakes early, ties on his apron, tucks his hair under a hair net, and prepares meals so that we have a freezer-full to choose from during the week. No matter the emotional challenge at work, I know I'll be calmed by the meals John has made with the talent of a master chef. Besides that, he possesses the know-how for preparing flavorful and filling dinners for much less than the cost to eat out. In the evening, John usually asks, "What should we have for dinner tonight?"

"You decide," is my typical response. I am terrible at making decisions, especially those involving food, a long-term side effect of anorexia. But the more I learn about PTSD, the more I understand that my decision dread has much to do with my anxieties around feeling out of control and in danger. Making even the smallest choices has become difficult. To eat a pear or a handful of nuts for a snack is like choosing between a total knee replacement or having a cortisone injection. Ironically enough, during the height of my anorexia years, choosing not to eat lent me a sense of control. But by letting

John decide what to eat for dinner, I am relinquishing that control. Because John knows about my history of anorexia, for the most part, he is willing to make the decision for me. But not always.

"There's still lasagna from yesterday," he'll offer. "Or I can take the coq au vin out of the freezer. You pick."

When John speaks in imperatives, I know it means he's mentally fatigued from a long day in meetings. The decision comes easily whenever we have coq au vin stored in the freezer. Simmered in red wine, and slow-cooked with caramelized onions and mushrooms, it's one of my favorite John dishes. And it's low in fat. Since he knows I prefer healthy foods, John uses dairy-free cheeses, unrefined sugars, and oil instead of butter in the recipes he has collected from his mother.

On most evenings, especially in the winter, we cuddle on the navy-blue sofa we bought as part of our new furniture collection after moving into the condo. We wrap ourselves in one of my mother-in-law's hand-crocheted afghans, and munch on popcorn while watching one of our favorite movies: *The Princess Bride*, *My House in Umbria*, *The Quiet Man*.

Instinctively, my right foot migrates toward John's left, and I rub my big toe against his sole. Without fail, he reciprocates and rubs his big toe against my sole. That's my favorite part of our movie nights.

Sometimes we play Irish music together during the evenings. He sits on the couch with his guitar, and I sit in the rocking chair with my fiddle. Because keeping time with music has always presented a challenge for me, he usually leads the tune or song: "One, two, tree," he counts, dropping the "h" in three like they do in parts of Ireland. I start playing after a couple of phrases, working the bow in time with the rise and fall of John's voice or the rhythm of his guitar picking. Sometimes we bicker over musical pitch.

"Melissa, your C is way off, too flat."

"Really?" For some reason, tunes in the key of C are my weak spot.

"Why don't we try a tune in a different key?"

"No, I like this tune. Let's try it again."

We play it again. And, again, I play a flat C.

John stops mid-tune. "Melissa, it's still off."

"I'll get it. Give me a little more time."

"Why don't you practice it later? Let's play a different tune for now."

"No. I told you I like this one."

I give it another try, then another, the C finally sounding like a C.

"That's it," John calls out. "Do it again."

And, again, we play the tune.

"John, wait. Now you don't sound right."

"Really?"

"Definitely off, way off."

John finger picks his guitar quietly, screwing up his mouth in concentration. "I think I have it now."

"It still doesn't sound right to me."

"Oh, I know what it is. My guitar is out of tune."

We have a standard list of tunes and songs we practice for the bimonthly music session John leads at a local pub. Since I've never played with experienced musicians before, during my first session, I sit next to John so I can hear his guitar. I've become used to his rhythm and don't want to be distracted by the eight other musicians sitting among us in the circle. The mix of instruments—penny whistles, mandolins, flutes, and bodhrans (Irish drums)—makes it that much more difficult for me to decipher each note. We each take turns choosing a tune, unlike a traditional session when one or two leaders start, and those who know it join in. Because there are thousands of Irish tunes, there are still many I don't know, so I sit back and listen for much of the session, my fiddle in one hand, the bow in the other, ready to jump in if someone plays a tune I recognize. When another fiddler starts playing my favorite, "Silver Spear," I look at John and whisper, "I know this one."

Bending the strings of his guitar, stamping his foot in time with the beat, he nudges me in the waist with his elbow.

I set the chin rest under my chin, wait for the beginning of the next phrase, and when it comes around, set the bow on the D string, move it back and forth, slowly at first, then faster. My fingers dance from one string to the next, connecting one note with another. The bow sweeps across the strings in long, light strokes, making legitimate music, music so sweet my lips and tongue tingle.

John nods at me and leans closer. "Great job, Hon."

I continue playing.

That moment is proof of the remarkable ways in which music can alleviate PTSD symptoms—a burst of happy, pain-distracting chemicals to the brain. The tingle now spreading down my shoulders, into my arms and legs, my toes and fingers, I rise slightly off the chair, as if I'm about to take off and fly into a secure atmosphere, a musical playroom where the tempo is steady, predictable, recognizable.

Between the spring and fall after John and I are married, walking becomes a tradition for us, too. We spend most Sunday afternoons in the Green Mountain Audubon Center in Huntington, where we hike the quarter-mile trail to Lookout Rock, and stop to sit on the wooden bench to take in the view of Camel's Hump. Sometimes my body appreciates a rest, as my healed back and pelvic injuries still ache like arthritic old-lady bones. "Melissa, do you see that?" is a question John inevitably asks each time we arrive at the lookout. He notices everything: a hawk dipping below a cloud, a patch of distant orange marking the onset of fall, a wild-berry plant peeking up from the earth.

As we ramble away from the lookout and deeper into the woods, John always takes the lead. No matter how many times we walk the trails, I cannot remember the way. "John, aren't we supposed to go that way?" I ask.

"No, Hon, follow me."

"Oh, yeah, now I remember."

In the fall, the varied-colored leaves carpeting the woods distract me, making me more confused about which trail to take. It's like looking through a kaleidoscope. I become dizzy, and pick my way through the woods, stepping carefully, one foot in front of the other. "You doing all right?" John asks every few minutes.

"Yeah, just taking my time."

Since the accident, clashing colors have become a new source of distraction and confusion. Because I can't think of any other reason for the change, I attribute it to PTSD. The accident has left me fearful of most things, including trees—one could crash down on us at any moment, cracking us in half. But John helps me approach them as if they are friends. "They're adjusting to the temperature change," he says one day while we're hiking along a trail, and I tell him the trees are moaning a lot and maybe we shouldn't be in the woods. "They're talking to one another, that's all."

As we trek on, I wonder if there is a way to translate the trees' moaning into human language. Maybe they are speaking to John and me. "Thanks for hanging out with us."

One summer, while walking through the Audubon, John becomes attracted to a cluster of five old maple trees. He points at a set of high branches, at a few leaves dangling like delicate earrings. "Look at them, Melissa. I can't believe they're still producing leaves." The trees must be centuries old, with the bark chiseled from wear and tear, the limbs covered in lichen and bent like forked lightning strokes. We decide to name them The Five Sisters, after deceased family members: Gert and Irene for both my grandmothers, Lucy and Eva for John's grandmothers, and Sasha for my cousin.

I walk up to Gert and run my fingers around the circumference of a rotted-out cavern in her trunk. As I lean into a solid section of the tree, I smell something friendly—a wooden chest stored with keepsakes. Gert, and her sisters, I believe, will stay standing for centuries more. They will not fall; they will not harm us.

When I turn away from Gert, John is running in circles, his arms outstretched, his gaze trained up toward the sky. "I'm gonna get it," he yells. "Here it comes." He reaches up higher, jumping up on his toes as it flutters and twirls, then drifts downward, straight toward him. "I got it." A maple leaf, red and green and whole, he holds in the palm of his hand.

"Your turn, Melissa."

I look up, wait for a leaf. When one starts floating downward, I skip, jump up, reach. I twist my body in the direction of the leaf, indifferent to the pain drilling through my back and hips, and lift my cupped hands toward it. It floats lower, lower, and at the last moment flies out of reach. So close. I whirl around in time to see another leaf, and snag it with my fingers. I catch it!

Like watching movies and walking in the woods, leaf catching becomes our tradition. Sometimes we bring one home and save it on a shelf in our living room. Sometimes we bring home a rock, a twig, an acorn. These small bits of nature we bring into our home extend the experience of being in the woods. It extends the experience of holding hope in the palm of our hands.

Chapter 42

Before the health department director has the chance to terminate me, I resign and accept a part-time position at a pediatrician's office. A month later, I ring in 2006 with one big bang—by giving an infant an incorrect vaccine.

I knock on my supervisor's door to tell her about the error. She doesn't answer. I knock again.

"Come in," Carol says, raising her voice above the rapid clicking of computer keys.

I turn the cold knob and open the door.

"What can I do for you?"

I tell her that I just gave the infant DTap—diphtheria, pertussis, and tetanus—instead of the vaccine I was supposed to give—DTap, Hepatitis B, and Inactivated Polio (IPV). She pushes back in her chair. The wheels skate along the plastic mat. She crosses her legs, uncrosses them, her stockings rubbing together like sandpaper.

"The vials are nearly identical," I say, offering what I believe to be a perfectly sensible response. "I'm sure other nurses have made the same mistake."

She gives me a pasted-on smile, the kind my mind reads as, "Good try but, no, none of the other nurses have screwed up such a simple task." To my great relief, she says she'll call the parents to let them know their child can receive the omitted vaccines during his next visit.

Leaving her office, feeling like a complete idiot, I torture my brain, trying to recall exactly what led me to screw up. *Melissa, you reached into the refrigerator, took out the green-and-black vial, the one with the black cap. Or was it the one with the green cap?* It isn't until I return to the medication room, empty vial in hand, when I realize I have given the incorrect vaccine. *It was the overhead lights. That's it. They must have caused a glare. That's why I misread the label.*

I can't recall ever giving an incorrect medication before. Maybe my mind's eye read the words on the vial in a disordered sequence. Maybe I'm missing more than I think I am: other medications I've administered but don't catch, bank account balances, credit card payments owed. And myself.

A few weeks into the job, a scheduled, thirty-minute physical assessment for a seven-year-old takes me an hour to complete. It takes me ten minutes just to measure her height. She steps onto the platform of the old-fashioned scale, and I ease the rod up over her head, the joint creaking as if it needs lubricating. I have to squint to see the six-point font numbers along the longitudinal axis. The longer I squint, the more the numbers appear to merge into a shapeless black glob. I step back to blink the film from my eyes, move in closer, and run my finger along the horizontal axis. I stop at the end of the rod, my finger now resting on top of a soft tuft of the little girl's hair.

"Okay," I assure her. "You can step off now."

I pencil a dot precisely at the thirty-three-centimeter mark on her growth chart, then look at it again to make sure I've plotted it correctly. It's an errant dot. Alone, like a distant planet, far below the other dots plotted at forty-one, forty-three, and forty-four. There are too many lines. Too many dots, like a pointillism painting. Too many numbers along the longitudinal and vertical axes, in inches and centimeters. Without thinking, I draw an X through my dot.

How simple is it to measure a child's height? Or a baby's head circumference and length? I measured those countless times in the NICU. Though my eyes were not injured in the accident, as with the numbers on the scale, when I wrap a measuring tape around a newborn's head, these numbers sometimes appear to be moving. My brain might as well be goat cheese. More than PTSD, there must be something wrong, way wonky wrong.

"How do you think things are going?" Carol asks during my three-month review.

"Pretty good," I blurt.

She draws a deep breath, exhaling quickly through her nose. I press my foot against the loose threads in the carpet, trying to push them back where they belong. She reminds me of my difficulties with measurements. "Yes, I know," I say. She also brings up my difficulty performing a rapid strep test. She doesn't need to remind me of this. How can I forget the seven-year-old who shoved his hand into my chest and pushed me away as I swabbed his throat with a Q-tip? All I got was a spot of saliva, not enough to run the test. Yes, I still remember Carol pulling his lower jaw down, then pushing the Q-tip into the back of his throat, his gag reflex so sensitive I thought he'd toss up that day's lunch and breakfast.

She then reminds me that I take too long assessing patients.

"I like to review things, you know, to be sure."

Another nose exhale.

I keep my mouth shut, afraid that whatever I might come up with will only affirm the dumb ass that I am.

Dr. Ulster, the pediatrician, is sitting in on the review. "People with anxiety feel the need to review things over and over," he says. From behind his cherry desk, he leans back in his chair, circling his thumbs. "PTSD is a form of anxiety."

Though I told Dr. Ulster about the accident and my PTSD diagnosis, I never showed him the PTSD specialist's letter; I worried he would have fired me. Moving from fear to anger, my fingernails piercing the cushion beneath me, I want to remind him that he is not my fucking therapist.

Because John and I need the money, I agree to a one-month extension of probation. But that April, as I sit on the same couch in Dr. Ulster's office, Carol asks, "Do you think this job might not be a good match for your skills?" Heavy rain pelts the window, spreading brown muck across the pane.

"I think I'm a good fit," I say, my voice weak. *Melissa, maybe you should stop now, before she says something you don't want to hear.* I sit up straight, my voice stronger. "I enjoy working with children. I work well with the staff."

Dr. Ulster slaps his knees, then stands up, his shoes scuffing the mat. "Let's meet in two weeks."

The slap is the trigger, and I'm four months in the past—the beginning of December—when I told John that Dr. Ulster offered me the job and I'd be starting in two weeks. But it would be part-time.

"Do you think we can manage?" John asked, since I'm the one who takes care of paying the bills.

"We'll figure it out," I said. Though I had no idea how, especially since I'd be working fewer hours and earning three dollars less an hour than at the health department.

Then, a week before Christmas, a letter arrived in the mail from the long-term disability company that had been paying me benefits for over two years. John paused from kneading dough, and looked over at me as I read, my face close to the fine print. The letter stated something about a maximum of twenty-four months coverage related to mental health issues like PTSD. *No. This can't be.* I tossed the letter across the counter.

"What do those fuckers have to say?" John asked.

When I told him what I've read, he stopped kneading and shoved his fist into the dough. "Those fucking bastards."

"I'm sorry." I covered my eyes so he wouldn't see me crying.

With the impending loss of $2,000 a month in disability payments, we had no back-up plan for how we'd pay the $1,100 a month mortgage on the condo, plus the monthly condo fee, the property taxes, two car payments, insurance, utilities, food, and the out-of-pocket expenses for my ongoing physical therapy and EMDR sessions.

"Hon, remember what you told me when you were offered the position? We'll figure it out." John wiped his hands on his apron and pulled me close to him, powdering me with maple sugar.

That May, I walk into Dr. Ulster's office, where he sits with his fingers steepled on the desk. "Have a seat," he says. I drop down onto the couch, sinking into the cushion. "Melissa, your performance is marginal."

I squirm, sinking lower. "I don't understand." None of the other nurses have said anything. "Can you explain?"

"We received an email from the parents of D.F. expressing dissatisfaction with your immunization technique. They observed you touching the sterile pad of the Band-Aid with your bare fingers." Dr. Ulster starts up with his thumb-twiddling, this time circling them fast, as if he's bored with having to keep dealing with my screw-ups.

Who is D.F.? I pick through my memory for a recognizable face or distinctive cry. The only patient I can think of is the toddler with a mop of vanilla-blond hair and a mean kick. It's the kick, and the cry I remember well. When I walked into the room during that second week of orientation, syringe in hand, he screeched like a howler monkey protecting its territory. Startled by his reaction, I almost screamed myself. As I so cleverly hid the syringe behind my back—too late—he buried his face into his mother's chest, tugging at her collar. Slowly, I walked toward him, and kneeled on the floor so that we were at eye level. He cried louder, snot dripping onto his upper lip, his chin, onto his mother's sweater.

"I'll stay and help hold him," she offered.

His mother laid him on the treatment table and crossed his arms over his chest.

"This is going to feel a little cold," I said, and sterilized his thigh with an open and ready-to-swipe alcohol pad.

His leg jerked, his knee missing my nose by centimeters. As I reached for the syringe on the table, he banged his legs against the mattress, and let out another shocking monkey screech. His mother looked at me, as if to say, "Let's get this over with." Pinning his legs down with my body, I counted the standard "One, two, three," then stuck him. The needle bounced off his taut skin. His mother glared at me. Quickly, I poked again. This time it went in. In then out. Blood oozed from his leg. I grabbed the gauze I had pre-opened from the packet, dabbed the injection site, and stepped back, out of nose-shot of his raised foot, his Light Up Sketcher positioned to kick-punch me straight in the face.

As I reached for the Band-Aid dangling from the edge of the examining table, he cried so hard he started hiccupping. "No - no - I - don't - want - that." Doing my best not to wince, I stuffed my hands in my pants pockets rather than letting his mother catch me plugging my fingers in my ears.

"I'll take care of it," she said.

I loosened the Band-Aid from the table and handed it to her. "Take your time," I said.

Stepping out of the examining room, I felt as if I were being accosted by glow-in-the-dark charts overflowing from a wall-mounted file holder, and a waiting room full of children with fevers, croupy coughs, and runny noses. And phones ringing, ringing, and ringing.

The EMDR specialist had written in her letter to my supervisor at the health department: "Moderate to severe anxiety when overstressed." I wanted to run from crying infants in the WIC clinic, and now I wanted to hightail it from colliding colors and nerve-jangling discord. But I needed Dr. Ulster to give me another chance. In the NICU, I was valued as one of the first to respond to a "code blue," and I was appreciated because I signed-up to care for the sickest babies. "I'll admit the twenty-four-week preemie." What if I just throw myself into the chaos? I thought. The ability to think and act fast would come back to me. Like riding a bicycle.

"Melissa, what do you think we should say to the family?" Dr. Ulster asks.

I say nothing.

"Well?" he persists, thumbs still whirling.

"I guess you should tell them that you spoke with me," though I'm still not sure if D.F. is the kicking monkey-howler. I don't ask if it is him, afraid that will only offer up more suspicion, yet another alleged incident of improper touching of a Band-Aid. "I did exactly as the other nurses showed me," I add, speaking louder, as if that will convince Dr. Ulster that I am right. Then a moment of doubt comes bashing down on my confidence. *Have I been touching the sterile part all along?*

Dr. Ulster continues. "I also received a phone call from parents who said they spoke with you on the phone, but you didn't follow-up with them, as you said you would."

"I don't remember that at all. Are you sure it was me?" He stares at me through his glasses, the forked vessel in his bird-like nose protruding.

Again, I rummage through my memory, this time going through all twenty-six letters in the alphabet, hoping that will elicit a certain name, even a distinct voice. But my brain fails me. Too many names and voices have come and gone since January, when I started training for telephone triage.

To help remember names and phone conversations, I take notes, lots of notes, and highlight phone numbers in yellow. Yellow, a reminder not to forget what you're supposed to do: "Return Stacey's call... check-in with Peter to see if Derek's asthma is under control... follow-up with Linda to make sure Dana is tolerating breastfeeding." I draw boxes next to the names of parents, then check the boxes after contacting parents. I even make it a practice to rehearse parents' names before calling. Still, I often get them wrong. Not Maggie but Marcia. Not Jason but Jonathan. I apologize to each parent, cross out the wrong name, then jot the correct one in capital letters, underline it, circle it. But the more I write, the worse my handwriting. I look at my notes and I'm unable to decipher what I've written. *Is that an M or an N? An eight or a three?* It's as if a different Melissa wrote those notes. "Can you clarify what you wrote here?" nurses ask me when following my shift. No, I cannot.

—

"Have you had trouble in the workplace before?" Dr. Ulster asks. I wonder if he knows about me nearly being fired from the health department; if so, who told him? He taps his pen against his palm, twirls it, round and round and round.

"No. Never."

"Well, that was before your accident," he says. *Your*, as if I owned the accident, as if it was my fault.

—

What if some time in the future I did own an accident? Replace a Buick LeSabre with my Subaru Outback. Replace Russell Weller with me. Put me behind the wheel, with my foot on the gas pedal instead of the brake, and I would have owned the accident. "Your accident" rings sharp in my ear, even now, all these years later. It hurts, the echo banging around in my head when I'm backing out of a parking space in a busy lot or driving in stop-and-go traffic or on a congested highway. Each time I learn of any driver confusing the gas pedal for the brake—a Texas teenager plummeting seven stories from a parking garage, or a sixty-four-year-old New Jersey woman leaving a car wash and plunging into a river—the slap of my real-life nightmare comes flying back at me: the bang of my body against the asphalt, the silence, everything black, then waking, terror-stricken and broken. I am reminded that it can happen anywhere, at any time, to anyone of any age—the motor vehicle turned lethal weapon. But that deadly day at the Santa Monica Farmers' Market was not *my* accident.

The computer on Dr. Ulster's desk buzzes, and a tiny button blinks repeatedly, with an incendiary light. He tells me he'll reduce my job responsibilities. I'll see to patients only: administering correct vaccines, measuring and plotting accurate heights, obtaining sufficient samples for rapid strep tests, all in an efficient manner. And no phone triage. But a reduction in responsibilities means a reduction in pay.

Chapter 43

JENNA.

Three years after the accident, flashbacks continue crashing into Jenna's life, preventing her from auditioning for acting roles. This is the end of her career, she thinks, and she'll be tormented by "these terrors every day for the rest of [her] life." Jenna wrote her first screenplay when she was fifteen, and landed a lead role in a 1987 episode of *Unsolved Mysteries*. In 1992, she appeared in *Buffy the Vampire Slayer*, about a young woman with superhuman senses who has the agility and speed to fight the forces of darkness. Since the accident, how is Jenna fighting the dark force of her panic? We're talking about a woman who was raised by teenage parents, who persevered through abuse, poverty, and an eating disorder. Jenna is not the type to give up. It will take many long years, but eventually she will slash the doubts growing wild in her rattled mind, and re-write the life-script of her dreams. Scene one: she'll become a published author of a story collection. Scene two: she'll get married. Scene three: she and her husband will venture on a year-long road trip across the United States. Scene four: Jenna will no longer suffer from traumatic flashbacks.

BARTLEY.

Bartley sustained a traumatic brain injury in the accident. A screenwriter and film director who founded Calgary's Lunchbox Theatre in 1975 and directed more than fifty plays, Bartley's recovery was complicated by what his doctors call "reduplicative paramnesia," a delusional belief that everything around him had been duplicated: his house, his car, even his wife of more than twenty years. Early on in Bartley's recovery, surgeons' hopes were slim at best that he'd regain his memory. But Bartley defied the odds, and his memory returned. Who knows how? Call it a miracle. Call it determination or faith. Or call it this (quoted straight from the *Calgary Sun*): "The other explanation is that I had horseshoes up my butt," said the doctor who performed Bartley's first critical brain surgery. Horseshoes or no horseshoes, Bartley would go on to produce a play, then perform himself in another play, *The Golden Hour*, a funny and inspirational one-man show about his fearless fight to regain his memory.

SHAMSI.

After six months in the hospital, one leg was shorter than the other, throwing Shamsi off balance. She could no longer wheel her cart through the Farmers' Market to buy fresh produce. Yet, she eventually did return to the market, this time wheeling along in her chair, greeted by farmers with gifts of oranges, lettuce, and squashes. Three years later, though, she still has not regained her balance, and is unable to stand at her kitchen counter to stir fresh tomato sauce or prepare fruit-filled desserts for her family. She sits at a table to slice fruits and vegetables, her fissured and seasoned black thumb proof of her culinary endeavors.

SANDRA.

A blues singer-songwriter, with an injured foot and dislocated shoulder from the accident, Sandra picks up her guitar and records the songs she has been nurturing for many months. Singing out loud, she voices her story of confusion, of love and pain, of magic and adventure. Three years after the crash, Sandra releases her CD, *Ghost Town Café*.

RUSSELL.

On January 5, 2004, the Los Angeles County District Attorney's Office charged Russell with ten counts of vehicular manslaughter with gross negligence. He pleaded not guilty to the charges before a Los Angeles Superior Court Judge, and was released on condition that he appear in court for all future proceedings. At a December 2004 hearing, he maintained his not guilty plea while his attorneys moved to dismiss the manslaughter charges, arguing he was a victim of "pedal error" causing sudden acceleration. Similarly, in the accident report issued by the National Transportation Safety Board, officials described what had happened as an "error in response execution," meaning Russell inadvertently accelerated when he intended to brake, and collided with the Mercedes Benz. Failing to detect his error, which the NTSB noted as "comparatively common," he unintentionally continued accelerating, launching through the market. His rising panic likely caused him to revert to the "habitual response" of pressing down harder on what he thought was the brake, but in fact was the gas pedal. Anyone, young or old, can commit pedal error. Still, Los Angeles Superior Court Judge Robert O'Neill denied the defense attorneys' request to dismiss the charges. "Hitting the gas pedal instead of the brake seems to me a clearly negligent act," he said.

Chapter 44

Sirens. Beeping horns. A bulldozer pushing rubble down a side street. We pass orange-and-white striped plastic barricades like the ones that came toppling down as Russell Weller sped down Arizona Avenue. I press my feet to the mat as John drives us through congested LA streets, then accelerates onto a six-lane highway toward Pasadena, where I will meet with Dr. Satz, a neuropsychologist who specializes in diagnosing and treating people with traumatic brain injuries—TBIs. My attorney, Mr. Archer, contacted Dr. Satz in the event the civil case he filed against the City of Santa Monica goes to trial. Nearly three years after the accident, in May 2006, I am relieved to know that there is someone who might be able to tell me why my brain cannot decipher vaccine labels, why I cannot measure heights accurately, why my brain overall is not getting the best gas mileage.

While initially hospitalized in California, I had multiple CAT scans taken of my brain, but none of them showed any obvious signs of bleeding or tissue damage, leaving the surgeons no reason for concern about a TBI. The psychiatrist at Cedars followed up with a screening. He asked me to count backwards by sevens from one hundred, to recall a list of words he mentioned ten minutes earlier, and to name as many animals as possible in sixty seconds. I passed. No one even mentioned the possibility of a TBI after that, until Mr. Archer arranged the appointment with Dr. Satz.

As John and I gain distance from LA, cars inch too close to our rear bumper. They speed past us, cut in front of us, crossing broken white lines. The cars are a smear of black, silver, and red. Soon, the surrounding landscape turns into green hills, and the snow-streaked San Gabriel Mountains draw closer as we leave behind the ache of orange-and-white.

Boutique shops and pink and purple hibiscus lining the sidewalks of Pasadena almost trick me into believing we're on vacation. (Other than splurging for our honeymoon in Ireland eighteen months ago, our frugal budget hasn't allowed money for vacations.) I envision us sleeping in late, then eating mushroom and spinach frittatas on the hotel's veranda overlooking Mediterranean style architecture. We'd browse the chic clothing stores, and John would convince me to try on a one-of-a-kind dress. "This would look great on you," he'd say. I'd try it on and twirl, the skirt spreading like a blossoming peony. In the evenings, we'd dine at a Spanish restaurant, listening to Flamenco dancers click their feet and clap castanets to Bolero music. For dessert, we'd dance, breast to breast.

My fantasized vacation with John pops like a balloon the following day, when we walk out of the sunlit spring morning and into the dimly lit stairwell leading to Dr. Satz's office. The wooden stairs sigh under the pressure of our feet. In the waiting room, a bookcase crowded with thick volumes of psychiatric books takes up the entire wall ahead of us. I step toward the bookcase, the wood luring me closer with its sweet-vanilla aroma, and run my hand along the worn spine of *Classic Cases in Neuropsychology*. I try to lift it off the shelf, but it's too heavy. It must be five hundred pages. *So many examples of us.*

The door leading to another room wheezes open. Dr. Satz walks toward us, wearing broken-in loafers, khaki slacks, and a cotton dress shirt with the top button undone. His casual style of dress surprises me. Neuropsychology, the study of the function of the brain and its relationship to behavior, conjures someone like Freud: pressed tie, starched white shirt, dark vest, and suit jacket. Dr. Satz shakes my hand. "Are you ready?" he asks, both of his hands now holding mine. "Melissa, this will be a long day for you. But we'll learn why you're experiencing so much difficulty at work." His unwavering voice reminds me of the promise the surgeon at LA General made to me nearly three years ago: *We're going to take care of you.*

I turn to John standing behind me. He nods as if to say, "It's okay, go ahead," but Dr. Satz waves us both into the room. "I want to ask the two of you some questions first." I wonder what he's going to ask John. "Can Melissa make a salad and pay attention to the water boiling on the stove at the same time?" No. "Does she go to the grocery store for milk, bread, and paper towels, then come home with milk, grapes, and eggs?" Yes.

John and I sit on a couch opposite Dr. Satz. John reaches out, and we squeeze hands.

"Melissa, what's the last thing you remember before you were hit?" Dr. Satz asks.

"The peach," I say, stretching my arm forward, the imaginary fruit cradled in my cupped palm. "I was holding a peach. Then it was gone. I heard a loud pop." My hands go for my ears. "I thought I got shot."

Dr. Satz shifts in his chair, crossing one leg over the other. "And what's the next thing you recall?"

"Doctors looking down at me." I pull my arms into my chest, as if I am cold. I feel so far away from the warmth outside: the sun's rays stroking palm-tree leaves, its butterscotch light dappling the horizon.

"Do you get fatigued and depressed?" he asks. "Yes, I get tired easily, especially when I have to do more than one thing at a time. I get brain fog." I admit I hate getting out of bed in the morning, that I'd rather stay beneath the covers than face another day of uncertainty. I curl my lips inward, as if I could take back my admission of those difficulties, difficulties I associate with inadequacy, unworthiness, with the notion that something is not only wrong, but it is somehow my fault.

"I see from your records that you did well as a student," Dr. Satz says. "You graduated from nursing school Magna Cum Laude."

A pause follows, a silence that's too loud. I want to fill it with something.

"Yeah, that's right." *But that was eighteen years ago. There's no way in hell the new Melissa can achieve Magna anything, other than Magna Cum Looser.*

I tell Dr. Satz that learning has become a monumental task since the accident. "I read the same passages from books over and over. It's frustrating." Sometimes I speak the sentences out loud, trying to capture each syllable and consonant. The next day, I can't remember the details of what I read, and have to go back several pages or an entire chapter. When watching a movie, the voices from the television sound like a record needle scratching across vinyl. The colors come at me too fast, like a spinning toy windmill. I ask John, "Can you pause the movie? I didn't see what just happened." It's as if my brain is a colander, impossible to fill.

Dr. Satz rubs his clean-shaven chin, murmuring indistinct, deep-thinking sounds that make me wonder if I am an outlier and he doesn't have much help to offer. He uncrosses his legs and drops a foot to the floor, the clunk of a heel startling me. "I don't know how you can work at all," he says. "What you described is not surprising for someone who has most likely suffered a head injury."

Oh, God, no. He did not just say that. Shit! Though I came to Dr. Satz to be evaluated for a brain injury, hearing it out loud makes it too real. And I'm not sure what this means for me, if I'll *ever* be able to work again, if John will feel the overwhelming burden, emotionally and financially, of caring for someone with so many needs. I glance at John and see that he is genuinely sad. I can see it in his drooped shoulders and sideways tilt of his head, the universal posture when someone is feeling grief. I also feel his sadness in the steady squeeze of his hand in mine.

Dr. Satz slides a piece of paper across the table, the crisp edge making the sound of a whisper, as if it hides a secret. He asks to speak with John, alone. "I'd like him to fill out this questionnaire, then I'll have you complete it." John lays his hand on my shoulder, his eyes misting. I know what he's thinking: *I'm on your side.* I learned to trust those words, and now interpret them to mean, "You're okay. I won't do anything to jeopardize your well-being."

"I want to get an idea of how John thinks you're doing," Dr. Satz says. Keeping the questionnaire in my line of sight, I walk backwards toward the door, reach for the knob, and turn back to glance at the questionnaire one more time before walking into the windowless waiting room. I feel like I just drank a double espresso; I can't keep still enough to sit. I pace to the tick of the grandfather clock hanging on the wall. Twenty minutes pass before Dr. Satz gestures me into his office. He pats John on the back, and asks him to take a seat in the waiting room.

On the table in front of me is a page listing various emotions and cognitive faculties. Dr. Satz asks me to rate them, one being the least problematic, ten being the worst. I imagine the numbers yelling at me, "You must choose." The first to be rated is "fatigue." Since I feel fatigued much of the time—first thing in the morning, after food shopping, after a half day of work, just thinking about work—I rate myself an eight. Fatigue makes me irritable. Time and again I tell John I'm not in the mood to be around people when he invites friends over. On nights when I go to bed early, while he watches classic cowboy movies, I trudge back into the living room to tell him to turn the volume down, because even the softest voice sounds like a fork scraping against a plate. I almost circle seven for irritability, but choose five, because I need Dr. Satz and John to see that I want to be inviting, likable, all things a well-behaved, good girl should be. God forbid I let anyone catch me in a bitchy mood.

I can't concentrate on a single task for a continuous amount of time without getting distracted. While poring over bank statements, trying to figure out how I managed to over-estimate the amount of money we have in our checking account, a glossy literary magazine on the coffee table will divert my attention and I'll skim through it. A five for "concentration" would be nice—at least average—but a six is more like it.

As for "word-finding capability," this time I have to go with a five. I often say to John, "It's on the tip of my tongue" when trying to come up with simple words like "spatula" or "tie." Since I can't recall scenes from movies the following day, or even a three-step cookie recipe five seconds after reading it, I go with a six for "memory." But, in all honesty, I am closer to a seven, probably an eight, maybe even a nine.

When John returns to the office, Dr. Satz places his evaluation and mine side by side on the table. Only a narrow strip of oak separates them. John and I look at one another's answers, then at each other, our mouths wide open. Most of our answers are either identical or nearly identical. John scored me higher for depression, word-finding, and memory than I did. I feel awkwardly exposed, stripped down naked.

That afternoon, I sit in a bare-walled room with Dr. Satz's assistant, answering questions that assess my level of executive functioning, the part of the brain that engages in complex thinking. I draw geometric figures from memory, forgetting which lines and angles belong where, rearrange blocks with various color patterns on each side, turning them over and over as I try to match up the patterns, and state as many words starting with the letter S as possible in sixty seconds. I name twelve. (The average thirty-something-year-old can name forty-three words.) I name faces and animals in photographs, and can't speak the word for a half lion, half human monolith reclining in a desert until prompted by the assistant.

"Sph …"

"Sphinx!"

Though I won't receive the results for a few weeks, I know my brain is broken. I know I will have to resign from Dr. Ulster's office. But I don't want to face Carol, Dr. Ulster, or my nursing peers in person. Instead, I call Carol the day after John and I return to Vermont.

"I won't be coming back. I can't."

"I understand," she says. She knew, too.

A few weeks later, I open the mailbox and pull out an envelope stamped with Dr. Satz's return address. I slide it to the bottom of the junk mail piled on our kitchen counter. John is at work; I want to wait for him to come home before I open it. I've anticipated the results of the testing to reveal a TBI, but don't want to be alone with them. I hold the envelope up to the light, daring to peek through, imagining what Dr. Satz has written: "Melissa is incapable of working as a nurse, ever again." But the envelope is too thick to see anything except sheer white. The immediate need to know gets the best of me. I can't wait for John. I slip my thumb under the flap. Push it up. Open. Tug the report from the envelope. I study all ten pages, every sentence, my eyes halting at three words that suck all the air out of me. "Substantial brain injury."

Seeing those words, smudge proof and unerasable, makes the diagnosis absolute, far more real than when Dr. Satz said out loud "head injury" during my appointment with him. It's easy to misinterpret when someone is speaking, but when typed in Times New Roman, there's no hiding. The truth has found *me.* Once again, I feel turned inside out, as exposed as when the EMDR specialist documented "PTSD is a chronic condition" in her letter to my supervisor at the health department, and again when I read John's ratings of my depression, word-finding capability, and memory. I want to believe Dr. Satz is wrong about what he wrote in the report: "Most cognitive recovery following a head injury takes place during the first two years." *I'm well past two years into my recovery.* His research might be outdated. But the truth is that words will not drip off the tip of my tongue, and I continue to forget the third task John asked me to do thirty seconds earlier. I continue to lose concentration while driving in traffic, and become distracted when boiling water for pasta. But after reading the latest research on brain injuries, I learn about neuroplasticity, the ability for brain cells to form new connections as a result of our interactions with stimulating environments, such as engaging in intellectual pursuits and social activities. Yes, I can, and will, come hell or high water, rebuild my brain.

Chapter 45

God, do I feel out of place in my stained clogs, worn jeans, and second-hand sweater, following Karin, the behavioral cognitive therapist, down the newly carpeted corridor toward her office, passing magazine quality photos of covered bridges and gold-leafed oaks hanging on pink walls. Then into her office, where stiff-spined textbooks on a shelf over her desk stand perfectly straight, like soldiers perpetually at attention. The desk itself is organized with a mug of tightly packed pens, the capped ends all facing up, and a squared stack of manila folders in the center, nothing on the inside sticking out.

As out of place as I feel, I know Dr. Satz wouldn't have suggested I travel ninety miles to Dartmouth Hitchcock Medical Center in New Hampshire if he didn't believe cognitive therapy would help. And it's November 2006, more than three years since the accident. If I am to succeed in any kind of work setting, or in life, my brain needs routine exercise to get back in shape, like CrossFit for brains. Driving all that way every two weeks to complete the six sessions better be worth it, even if it means sleeping all afternoon when I get home, then going to bed early and sleeping until 10:30 the next morning.

During the first session, Karin opens a binder as thick as a coffee-table book. But rather than inspiring photos, each page is filled with instructions on managing day-to-day exercises for people with a TBI. She calls the exercises Memory and Attention Adaptation Training, or MAAT. It sounds more like a new discipline program for poorly-trained old dogs.

She hands me the binder. I stare at the shiny surface, at the reflected silhouette of my face, then open it and begin reading to myself: "It is estimated that upwards of 1.5 to 2 million Americans each year suffer from some type of TBI. Most TBIs, between 50% to 80%, are considered to be mild, traditionally defined as a blow to the head with loss of memory after the injury (or post-traumatic amnesia)."

The statistics scroll through my mind like a ticker tape. "Fifty percent to eighty percent are considered to be mild." I finger the edges of the sharp page, sharp enough to give you a zinger of a paper cut. My head hit the pavement when I fell to the ground at the Farmers' Market. A blow to the head. I suffered from post-traumatic amnesia for several hours. No amnesia for weeks or months. No loss of consciousness for greater than twenty hours, all indicators of a moderate to severe TBI. *I must have sustained only a mild injury.* I'm confused, though; Dr. Satz suggested I sustained a "substantial" injury.

"Karin, I don't understand. How could my injury be as bad as Dr. Satz said if I didn't lose consciousness for too long? And, yes, I had amnesia, but it didn't last more than a few days."

"It's not always that clear-cut," she says. "It appears that you sustained a mild TBI, but that doesn't mean the consequences are mild."

I understand the CAT scans showed no bleeding or neuron fiber damage, and I scored high on the Glasgow Coma Scale—a fifteen-point scale used to measure eye-opening, verbal, and motor responses in trauma patients. But I'm now doubting Karin's explanation. Do I have a brain injury? Or do my symptoms mean I am just plain stupid? The denial channel is playing in my head like catchy background music. I have to ask, "Exactly what kind of consequences?"

"Think about the difficulties you've had in the workplace," she says. "That's what I mean. Sometimes it's not until someone's cognitively challenged that the symptoms become apparent."

Apparent to whom? The denial channel turns up full volume. My inability to multi-task, the blurring of words and numbers on the page, the chronic fatigue were not apparent to the health department director. She saw me as symptomless when she declared, "You're not fulfilling your job description." My coworkers see me as someone who appears perfectly fit, who doesn't look as if she has been hit by a car. It's alarming to consider that I have a TBI, and yet I'm the only one who notices.

My new diagnosis gives me a free, lifetime membership to an ever-growing group of survivors whose injuries are commonly referred to as "invisible," injuries that are neither seen nor felt by others.

I continue reading through the binder Karin gave me. "Complaints about memory and attention are common. In individuals with mild injury, these symptoms usually clear up in days to weeks, although in about ten to fifteen percent of people, these symptoms can persist for months or even longer."

I point to the sentence about symptoms persisting, and ask Karin how long I should expect mine to last.

"That's difficult to know," she says, holding open her empty palms.

I'm going to TBI jail, and I don't know how long I'll be in?

I turn to the next page, where a chart lists how often people with TBIs experience specific attention and memory problems. Forty percent forget appointments and about fifty percent forget the content of daily conversations. I flip ahead to a page where another chart lists how frequently those without a brain injury suffer from memory lapses. Twenty-seven percent forget why they entered a room. "Keep in mind that minor memory problems are part of everyday healthy living," the section before the chart notes. I wonder what the research means by "minor." Forty percent? Twenty-seven percent? Where does minor end and significant begin? I anticipate what John would say. He'd be honest but gentle, God bless the sweet guy that he is. "Honey, I'm sorry, I wish I could say differently, but you probably forget details of a conversation more than most people."

Karin then introduces me to an Activity Schedule Form. The days of the week are printed vertically across the top of the page and the hours horizontally along the left margin, with stark white spaces in the middle waiting to be filled in.

"Really?" I ask her. "I never needed a date book before." Before the accident, I never missed paying a bill, and easily memorized my inconsistent nursing schedule. I was even better than the average person at remembering birthdays and anniversaries. I don't know what to assign to the cluster of blank squares. Each one is the size of a pillbox, too compact to fit any haphazard life into.

"You can use this form to mark mealtimes and remind yourself to take your medications," Karin says.

"I'm not sure I need that." I'm taking only three medications: Celexa to temper my anxiety, Trazadone to lift my depression, and Ritalin, a stimulant to kick my brain into high gear so that I can stay on task.

"It can't hurt to try," Karin encourages.

Sometimes it's 11:00 in the morning before I remember to eat breakfast, or 1:00 in the afternoon when I realize I have not brushed my teeth. I don't tell Karin that I sometimes can't remember if I've taken my Ritalin. Sometimes I skip taking it. Other times, I count the remaining pills for the month to be sure I have not doubled up on the dose. God help me if I miscount. My heart would bolt through my chest like a spooked horse. After our first meeting, I decide to fill in those squares: eat, take meds, do stretches, nap, practice fiddle—and call Dad. Those squares, and later a date book, become extensions of my brain.

During my next visit with Karin, she teaches me how to play what she calls "the name game." When you meet people, you repeat their names back to them. "Hi Margaret. It's nice to meet you, Margaret. Hope to see you soon, Margaret." Over the Christmas holiday, John and I attend parties for the Rotary Club and the American Lung Association, where he works as a fundraiser, and he introduces me to several people. I shake their hands, look them in the eye, and smile. "Nice to meet you, Diane. Nice to meet you, Jason." Seconds later, their names vanish. "I whisper to John, "What's her name? Debbie? What's his name? Josh?"

As we leave each event, others say, "It was nice to meet you, Melissa."

"It was nice to meet you, too" (person whose name I forget).

John is the middle child of eight siblings. When I first met them, I repeated each name in my head, but they dissipated like vapor. I remembered their names only after seeing each sibling again and again, after repeatedly hearing the nuances of each voice. It's the identifying features—the timid voice, the wandering lazy eye, the thick eyebrows—that lock the name in place, help me hold onto that person.

While at a party early on in his recovery after the Farmers' Market accident, Bartley didn't recognize a single guest, people he knew before his injury. It wasn't until months later, after his wife showed him photos from the gathering, that he recognized most of the faces. While at the party, if Bartley didn't know who his friends were, what did he say to them? Maybe he said, "It's great to see you, too."

During the last visit with Karin, she teaches me the "method of loci," or the "memory walk," a form of mental note taking where you visualize images to remember things like groceries. I'm not sure what prompts these images, but a pound of green beans propped on my head comes to mind, as do a loaf of rye bread tucked into my bra and a quart of milk cradled in my arms. In the past, if John asked me to get a few items at the store, maybe angel-hair pasta, red peppers, and raisin bran, I'd walk up and down the same aisle three times trying to find pasta. I'd pick up a box of corkscrew pasta, then put it back. I'd pick up another box—spaghetti—toss it into the cart. I'd wander the aisles for nearly an hour, the bright lights, like those in the WIC clinic, making my eyes cross. I'd make my way to the cereal aisle. Fruity Pebbles. Frosted Flakes. Froot Loops. Too many colors. Too many designs and cartoon characters. Finally, I'd pluck a box of oat bran cereal from the shelf, walk down the aisle toward the registers, passing the dairy section, walking faster through refrigerated air, even faster past the meat department, shivering at the gross thought of raw chicken flesh. I had never needed a shopping list for three items.

"We needed angel hair," John would remind me when I returned home from the store, his hands buried in a mixing bowl of seasoned ground turkey. "We never eat spaghetti." He'd blow off his frustration with a groan, then soften and tell me not to worry. "I'll get it, Hon." He'd rifle through the grocery bag, rustling the paper. "Did you happen to get the peppers?" I'd throw my hands in the air, pissed at myself for forgetting. "I'll be back in a few," he'd say, and give me a soft kiss on the cheek before dashing out of the house.

At the grocery store, a few days after my final visit with Karin, I imagine spinach leaves waving at me from the crisper, sweet cherry tomatoes in the rocking chair, and a box of Goldfish crackers sitting next to me on the couch. It works.

Chapter 46

"I signed up for a class," John says when he calls from work one day. For months, John has talked about returning to school. The evening before, while the two of us were lying in bed listening to the tree frogs croak during an unusually hot Memorial Day, he mentioned it. "Go for it," I said.

I want to say his returning to school inspires me, and it does. But I won't deny it; I'm envious. Since resigning from Dr. Ulster's three years ago, I've worked as a school nurse, a receptionist for a nonprofit, and an infusion nurse for a medical supply company. Chronic back pain, anxiety, and fatigue drove me to quit each of those jobs. Now, a few months unemployed, I am spiraling into a dark funk, and can't seem to get out of my own way. I need to find something useful to do soon, something that makes me feel like I'm succeeding.

I hang up with John, and decide I can use a nap. I walk into the bedroom, and as I'm about to crawl beneath the afghan, I notice the top drawer to the file cabinet next to my side of the bed is partially open. I hip-check the drawer packed with page after page of medical records, legal documents from my attorney, and the black binder overstuffed with articles and other paraphernalia from the accident. It pops back open, and right there, face up on top of the binder, is the notebook I used as a journal during the early days of my recovery. I can't remember the last time I looked through it. I lift it out from the cabinet, and run my hand along the laminated gold cover embossed with the word "Trust" in deeper gold calligraphy. The letters slant to the right, as if a breeze were blowing them forward into the future.

I thumb through the notebook, pausing at the third page where I had written "things to look forward to: walks in the woods, playing fiddle, independence." On the next page, in black marker, I copied from John Steinbeck's *East of Eden* the Hebrew word *Timshel*—meaning thou shalt—a command. I recall a favorite passage from the novel, where Lee disagrees with this translation, and argues instead for "thou mayest," implying free choice. Like John, I can choose to take the class, too. But as I do when faced with making most choices, I fret over whether I should sign up, not even knowing anything about the class. I trace my fingers over *Timshel*, trying to feel my way toward a decision.

I drop the journal to the floor and call John back. "What's the class about? What's on the syllabus? When does it start?"

"It's Global Issues in the Media. We'll be researching and writing about worldwide topics. Why don't you sign up?" The last time I took a class for a grade was in nursing school, and that was twenty years ago.

"I'll have to think about it," I say. Overthink is more like it. My head goes wonkers, turning and turning like one of those fidget spinners. I'd be the slowest in the class. I'd be asked to drop the class. Or I'd finish with a big fat F.

I stare at the journal lying there on the floor. "Trust, trust, trust," I speak out loud, then pick it up and open it to the one dog-eared page where I logged part of a quote from the writer Richard Bach: "There are no mistakes."

I sign up for the class.

Two evenings a week, for six weeks, John and I sit among a group of mostly twenty-year-old students, discussing the Israeli-Palestinian conflict, peak oil, and the wars in Iraq and Afghanistan. By now, I've come around to the idea of using a date book, and fill in each day of the week with "Homework, 10:00 a.m. to noon." While reading the assigned books, I mark the margins with notes and tab the pages with yellow sticky notes. When not reading, I am writing. By the end of the six weeks, we are expected to complete a research paper on climate change, a news article on universal health care, and a short story. Between reading and writing, I nap. After finishing my homework each day, I nap again.

When we hand in our first paper, I'm worried sick, about-to-vomit sick. *Is my argument for universal health care strong enough? Did I cite my sources correctly? Did I correctly format all quotes?* I prepare for the worst. I know for sure John will get an A. He writes poetry that would wow Pablo Neruda. How humbled I still am with the memory of the poem he wrote for me soon after our first date: "Out to the west, to guzzle and wander the old Spanish sun. To the market she passes, and dances the stalls. And the daisies and ivy and sugarcane call. And lifting the peach to the shine of her face, she misses the moment when death rattle roars."

We both receive an A on that first paper; we both complete the class with an A. My mental funk starts to lift. My fear of failing, of pissing someone off, of agonizing over every little dumb detail has become a pummel horse. I will vault over it.

Chapter 47

It isn't until August, a month after the class ends, before I have it in me to take that long-legged leap—back to the file cabinet. I open it, this time all the way, and pull out the black binder. It's heavy, like a slab of granite, but that doesn't stop me from lugging it to the dining room table. I am now ready to take a close look at what's inside. As I open it, letters, the disabled parking placard with the wheelchair symbol, the plane ticket from California to Boston, all tumble to the floor. I pick up the placard, surprised to see it has not faded at all; it's as bright red as the day I received it in the mail six years ago.

"The binder is how you put your life back together," a friend told me earlier that summer. "It's how you put *yourself* back together." I look away from the binder and see the old Melissa doing CPR on a baby, running for miles along sandy roads, and skiing shapely S turns through endless powder. But those images quickly flick to scenes of a Melissa going for a short walk, then falling asleep on the couch when she gets home. An old fiddle, its spruce body without its pristine finish, the cracks in its tailpiece wide and jagged, the surface marred with fissures. What would the fiddle look and sound like if the cracks could be repaired? Seductive? Breathy?

I turn the pages, fanning dust motes from the plastic protectors, and stop at a newspaper photo of a woman reclining stiffly in a chair by her hospital bed: eighty-nine-year-old Shamsi. Her neck is wrapped in a thickly padded brace, and her legs and feet are dressed in white bandages. She looks like a wooden doll with pointed toes and long-carved fingers and legs. If you bent her from the waist, even slightly, she'd snap in half.

After the accident, I didn't want to look at Shamsi's photo or at any of the photos laid out "above the fold" of newspapers. Nor did I want to read the articles. I skimmed through some of them, the ones with no photos, before tucking them in the binder in my bedroom closet at Kathleen and Rick's. Now, I hold the binder open for a long time, my face close to Shamsi's photo, as if I don't want to miss anything, not the V-shaped crevices in her cheeks, the port-wine bruise on the right side of her forehead, the brace supporting her neck, the raw gouge on her left calf where surgeons excised muscle and skin to cover the bones jutting out from her right leg.

I wince, picturing her bones crunching on impact, the gash spreading across her cheek, her right ear ripping in half, her temporal artery rupturing. She was standing near Second Street when the Buick hurtled through the market. I was between Second and Third Streets. How close was I to Shamsi, Shamsi to me? Inches? Feet? Who came to her aid? I imagine her screams for help—pushing all the air out against her brittle ribcage—then a rescue worker hooking a red tag around her toe. That red tag was her pass to twelve hours of surgery, where doctors inserted steel plates into her broken neck. The red tag was her pass to six months in the hospital.

Like me, Shamsi was a caretaker: for her mother who had suffered a stroke, for her son who had died of cancer, for her sister who had a brain tumor, and for her husband afflicted with Alzheimer's. I need to know more about her, the woman who once lay so close to me, maybe only an arm's reach away.

I search the Internet for her address and phone number, computing the math in my head: *If she was eighty-nine in July 2003 and now it's August 2009, she must be ninety-five.* I have no idea, though, if she's still alive, or what I would say if I were to call her. "Have you healed? I read that you used to go to the Farmers' Market every week and that you've been back since the accident. What was it like? Do you still shop for tomatoes?" I stare at the computer, at her phone number, the screen in focus, then out of focus. I rub my eyes, but that doesn't change anything. Thin blue lines shimmy inward from all four sides. I pick up my cell phone, poke the three, pause, poke the one, the five, and quickly dial the remaining numbers. In rapid succession, a series of faraway rings echoes, like calling someone overseas.

"He—he—hello?"

"Yes, I'm looking for Shamsi."

The woman speaks a jumble of foreign vowels, then, "Who? No Shamsi. Who do you want?"

My throat is so dry I almost can't speak. "Sorry. I'm looking for Shamsi?"

She speaks loud and fast, sputtering lots of wet P's and S's. Then nothing.

I wonder if I dialed the wrong number. Or had Shamsi died, and I upset a family member by calling and asking for her? I quickly dismiss that thought, and reason that the person who answered couldn't understand me, because I pronounced Shamsi's name incorrectly. I want that to be the truth. If she had died, I'll now never be able to ask her if she thinks of Russell Weller when she looks at her scars, or feels a sting in her right ear, a throb in her hip, an ache in her leg. Or if she thinks of Russell Weller each time she reaches for an ugly tomato.

That same day, I type her a letter:

August 17th, 2009

Dear Shamsi,

Hi. My name is Melissa Cronin. I was also injured at the Santa Monica Farmers' Market when Russell Weller sped down Arizona Avenue. I saw your photo in *The Los Angeles Times* and read the 2003 article about your injuries and part of your recovery. I'd like to know how you're doing now. If you're willing to talk, please call or write.

I mail the letter, wondering if she moved, and I'll never hear back. After a day or two, I Google her name again, and click on a *Los Angeles Times* article dated September 16, 2006. "Shamsi Khani, ninety-two, the oldest victim of the 2003 crash dies. The popular regular had defied slim odds of survival."

I lay my forehead against the keyboard. *If I only reached out to her sooner.* If only. But I do make a virtual visit to her gravesite. The website of Mount Sinai Memorial Park in Los Angeles shows a photograph of her granite gravestone flush against the cemetery's green grass. Contained within a bronze border is her epitaph: "Shamsi Maman Khani. The symbol of love—our shining light. Beloved matriarch, mother, grandmother, and great-grandmother." Next to her epitaph is an etching of an eternal flame.

Shamsi made her final trip to the market a week before she died. Instead of purchasing tomatoes, she chose Asian pears, symbolic of comfort and peace.

Maybe that's how she put herself back together, by returning.

Now that I've brushed the dust off the binder, opened it, and let myself in, it's as if I've walked into a museum that has been closed for the past six years for renovations. I want to walk around in there and explore more of its valuables. Tucked in the inside pocket of the binder is a manila folder stuffed with five-year-old legal documents my attorney sent me. I spread them across the living room floor, tossing aside lengthy and obtuse legalese in search of the names of the injured, the families of the dead, and the attorneys involved in the civil case against the City of Santa Monica. There must be twenty attorneys' names.

I Google each name and find fifteen of the attorneys. I type an email to the first one on the list:

> Dear Mr. Whitman,
> I was injured at the Santa Monica Farmers' Market accident in 2003. I am ready to write about that horrific day and its aftermath, and would like to speak with other survivors. I know this may be emotionally difficult for some, if not all, so I'm only asking if you could forward my contact information to your clients.

I drag the cursor to the send button, pause, my hand trembling over the mouse, the cursor vibrating in tiny circles. *Won't they be too busy representing clients to answer me?* I worry the email sounds too desperate, or not desperate enough. I press send.

A few days later, I receive an email from Sandra. Her attorney must have forwarded her my contact information.

> Hello Melissa,
> I have also written about that day which lasted many years for many people, and for others who are still recycling their trauma. We all process differently. I am also writing about my recovery. That was my shoe that ended up on top of Mr. Weller's car. The writing I am working on now is more about the journey of working through trauma. The CD I wrote, "Ghost Town Café," was partly inspired by that.
>
> La Musicas La Medicina,
> Sandra

Though I've recently read about her in old news blurbs, and looked at her website after researching her name, receiving Sandra's email makes her real. I open Sandra's attached document, titled "Requiem for All Between Earth and Sky":

> How do we speak the language of blood and spirit? How do we utter words of life and death in the same breath? I am watching the spirits of the dead ascend into the sky. The fruit, ten minutes before arranged as if in a still life, lies splattered around me. Two bystanders are helping me. Bless them. My left foot is oozing blood. My left arm is broken. I know immediately I am conscious. I am alive, in shock. I review in my mind what happened. I hear the sound of an explosion. I turn around. There's a car traveling at the speed of darkness thirty feet away, bearing down on me.

I remember the moment before daylight turned black. The peach in my palm. *Pop.* Quick and deafening.

As I did with Shamsi, I need to know more about Sandra. We share so much in common: the pyramid of fruit, the sound of an explosion, music. In the Google search bar, I type as fast as my fingers will move. "Sandra Bacall."

Photos of her grace her website's gallery. One of them shows Sandra, a forty-something-year-old wearing a teal-and-white sundress and tall black boots. She's crouched low to the grass, her long auburn hair swept forward, her blunt bangs shielding her forehead like window blinds. She holds the neck of her folk guitar over her shoulder, the hourglass body proudly displayed like a trophy, while she looks at the camera with deep-set eyes. Her chin is slightly lifted in confidence. I get the impression that she's a soothsayer who predicts only the best of outcomes.

I continue searching through her website, and find the page where it reads, "Her famous shoe ... on top of the old man's Buick." Though she mentioned the shoe in her email, it doesn't resonate until now. Her lost shoe. My lost sneakers. We share that, too. After searching the Internet for article after article, looking for Sandra's shoe, I find it. A black sandal with a wedge heel, standing upright on the roof of the Buick. Intact.

There are many more lost shoes among the seventy-three of us, and sometimes I envision them amassed in a landfill, molding together within the Earth's solid core, each one taking a thousand years to decompose.

Chapter 48

Grim-lipped, tangled eyebrows, vacant eyes magnified by metal-rimmed glasses, pouches beneath the eyes like used tea bags—Russell Weller's photo.

An early October chill whisks through the cracked-open balcony door as I leaf through the black binder searching for news reports about Russell Weller. I stop at an article with that photo taken three years ago, September 2006. He had just arrived at the Clara Shortridge Foltz Criminal Justice Center in Los Angeles for the beginning of his trial.

It's hard to look at him, wondering what turmoil lived inside him as he anticipated the outcome of the case. I shift my full attention to an article written on the day after the crash. "I couldn't believe what I was seeing," a bystander reported. "He was hitting people and they were flying. When he hit someone, you could hear it. Boom! Boom! Boom!" Hot blood surges to my head. I push the binder aside, go to the kitchen, and pour myself a glass of water. *Boom, boom, boom* reverberates between my ears with each swallow. I go back to the binder, but decide not to finish reading the article, and skip to the next one. "How many people did I hit?" the reporter quoted Russell Weller saying after he stepped out of the Buick. "If you saw me coming, why didn't you get out of the way?" My face stings, as if Russell Weller himself just slapped me. I wonder why someone who just drove into a crowd of people would ask such a thing. From shock? If I could answer Russell Weller right now, I'd ask him, "How could any of us have gotten out of your way? You were speeding, at sixty miles an hour." I clap the binder shut and consider shredding every single article stamped with Russell Weller's name and photo.

But if I want to empty myself of the accident—the rumbling *boom, boom, boom*—I must continue reading to try to find words that will explain what happened, and maybe ease my resentment toward him. More than that, I need to try to forgive; the attempt alone will at least maintain my "good" status, the one who's always inclined to give others the benefit of the doubt. To forgive, though, I still need to figure out who is really to blame: Russell Weller, for not listening to his wife when she asked him to let the postman take the letter when he came to pick up the mail. His family, for not taking his keys away. Or the City of Santa Monica, for failing to protect pedestrians with roadblocks sturdier than flimsy orange-and-white striped plastic barricades. Not for the first time, I mull over forgiveness. Isn't forgiveness like emotion? A state of mind dependent on one's mood at the time. One day you might forgive, the next day you might say, "This is bullshit."

"He can't be a nice guy," John says that evening when I share with him what Russell Weller said at the accident scene: "Why didn't you get out of my way?"

"John, he could not have meant what he said. He panicked."

More opinions from articles I read ricochet through my head like bullets. "I know it wasn't an accident... he did it on purpose... he hit everything he could... coward... murderer."

To bystanders, these reactions were not far-fetched. The speed at which Russell Weller was driving and accelerating might lead anyone to believe he was a murderer—a terrorist whose aim was to kill as many people as possible, even if it meant risking his own life, too. The aftermath of the heinous crime resembled a war zone, with the chorus of screams, the trail of bodies, the helicopters circling overhead. The Santa Monica Farmers' Market crash came two months shy of the second anniversary of 9/11. Americans were still reeling from the worst attack on U.S. soil.

But Russell Weller was not a murderer. He did not leave his house that morning scheming to kill people.

John's eyes water. "I can't imagine how painful it would be if it was my old dad who was driving." I can't imagine if it was my dad, either.

Chapter 49

Nearly a year after the accident, while visiting my father and his wife at their summer home, she spurts anger toward Russell Weller, saying he should go to jail. My father sits silently across from me at the kitchen table, his glossed-over stare fixed out the window on some point far off into the distance. My chest rises and falls with heaviness. I look out the open window facing the ocean, watching it wash up against the shore, listening for each crash against the rocks. My father and I are both staring at some truth held in the crest of a wave.

A few months after that visit, my father sends me a copy of a letter he mailed to farmers' markets throughout the country. "The accident may have been prevented if appropriate safety measures were taken, such as the placement of barricades. The Santa Monica Farmers' Market massacre will come back to haunt us if we do not take immediate measures."

As I read the letter, I believe my father's words. I believe he wrote the letter because he needs to know he has acted to effect change, to protect his daughter and others from potential future harm.

Behind my father's glossed-eyed stare, between the lines of his letter, I read this: "It's not me! I'm not an old man. It will never happen to me. I'm a perfectly good driver."

He *was* a good driver. Then Alzheimer's creeps in and begins to wreck his brain. The dings and dents to all four sides of his car tell the story. It's nine years after the accident when I am handed an opportunity Russell Weller's family never took: to intervene before people died. For me, that means taking the keys away from my seventy-two-year-old father. Fear of my father stalls me. Doubt stalls me. At first, I wonder if I am over-reacting, and that maybe he is telling the truth: The dings and dents are the fault of other drivers banging into his car as they pull into the small square parking lot of his office building. *Dad drives only during the day. He's not Russell Weller. Why not let him drive locally, to the grocery store, to his favorite Italian restaurant?* But Russell Weller lived less than a mile from the post office.

When my father's Alzheimer's worsens, I have to do the right thing. I ask his neurologist for a letter stating that he should not be driving, then send it—along with his medical records—to the Department of Motor Vehicles. "I know it was that fucking doctor's fault, whatever his name is," my father screams the day he calls me to say he has received a letter from the DMV informing him that his license had been revoked. It tears my heart in two when he sobs on the phone like I've never heard him sob before. "If I can't drive," he cries, "I'll die. I swear, I'll die."

I don't know what to say. But I know what I feel. I feel like a liar, a cold-hearted coward for not admitting to him it is my doing, my fault. It takes time, but knowing others are safer with him off the road helps me to forgive myself. What comforts me even more is the group of home health aides who look out for my father. He is among the few who can afford long-term care insurance, which pays for caregivers to be in the home twenty-four-seven. They drive him to his favorite Italian restaurant, to the bank, or to his office, where he rifles through business contracts, and plays the part of a once-upon-a-time real-estate developer. He eventually enjoys having his caregivers do the driving, and as he becomes comfortable with them bathing and dressing him, he stops feeling around in his pockets for his car keys.

How much easier it would have been if he gave up driving on his own. How much easier it would be if we all were as acquiescent as Prince Philip. The prince willingly gave up his license in the wake of the 2017 crash, when the ninety-seven-year-old's Land Rover collided with another car carrying two women and a nine-month-old baby.

But Prince Philip is an outlier. The truth is that the burden often falls on families, and they're not always capable of dealing with the challenge of taking the keys away from their aging parents. We need sensible solutions, similar to measures adopted in other countries, most notably Japan. As one of the fastest aging nations on Earth, Japan saw the number of older drivers increase from nearly 8 million in 2003 to roughly 20 million in 2023. Add to this the slew of fatal traffic accidents in Japan caused by drivers seventy-five and older. The government could no longer ignore the inevitable and had to act. Their response was immediate: those who are seventy-five and older must undergo dementia screening. Those age seventy and older are required to participate in driving-instruction classes and lectures, followed by a test drive with a police officer. For some drivers, this is the moment I imagine they dread most, when the officer advises that it's time for them to retire from driving.

Yes, the call for age-appropriate testing may stink of ageism, but when it comes to hearing, vision, and reaction time, change is incontestable. So why not at least make eye exams routine, say every three years for drivers seventy and older? This is the solution a widower from the United Kingdom proposed to the country's Secretary of State for Transport. For him, the matter was painfully personal. In 2012, his wife was tragically killed when an eighty-two-year-old driver confused the gas pedal for the brake. The car was traveling fifty-four miles an hour when it hit her. Her husband and two-year-old son were there. They saw it happen—their nightmare—up close and real.

The Secretary of State now requires drivers seventy and older to renew their licenses every three years. However, drivers are responsible for notifying the Driver and Vehicle Licensing Agency of any medical conditions, such as vision impairments, that might affect their ability to drive safely. As in the U.S., the U.K. does not legally enforce the reporting of medical conditions. They have essentially left it to families to carry the full burden when it comes to taking away the keys. Straight from the first paragraph of the GOV.UK webpage page titled Voluntarily Surrendering Your Driving License: "There's no legal age at which you must stop driving. You can choose when to give up or surrender your license and for how long, whether your reason is a medical condition or something else."

But what if you're iron-willed, and refuse to stop driving, even if you've killed people? Like seventy-four-year-old Stella Maychick. In 1992, she raced through two stop signs when she confused the gas pedal for the brake and killed five people in Washington Square Park. After her license was suspended for "failure to use due care," she applied to have it re-instated in 1994. She failed the driving test—for running a stop sign. She re-applied for her license again in 1995. This time she passed, and drove for several more years. How fortunate that she did not run more stop signs.

I wonder what I'll do when I'm old, and my arthritic, tired foot is unable to move fast enough from the gas pedal to the brake as the driver ahead of me stops short to let pedestrians cross. I hope I do what is right and safe—cut up my license, toss my car keys into the trash. But it's not so simple for everyone; there are many more Stellas out there. Especially for those living off the grid, in the middle of nowhere. How do they get to a far-away medical appointment or grocery store, or visit a friend, if the nearest bus or train station is ten, fifteen, twenty miles away? Judith, the eighty-nine-year-old woman I cared for as a wellness nurse, and whose family eventually did the right thing, ended up spending much of her lonely time at home. It terrifies me to think of what will come of me as I age, if I will face the same fate as Judith, socially isolated, scared, and alone.

Chapter 50

More articles about Russell Weller, dated November 2006:

> A judge attacked George Russell Weller's "enormous indifference" and "unbelievable callousness" in running down and killing ten pedestrians in a Santa Monica open-air market. "The eighty-nine-year-old deserved prison for his crime," the judge said... "but because of and only because of his rapidly declining health, I will place him on probation."

I clutch the page, and continue reading: "Weller has never once expressed in court any remorse for his actions. I will never understand his stubborn and bullheaded refusal to accept responsibility, to put this matter to rest for everyone, including himself."

Due to his declining health, Russell Weller was not present in the courtroom to hear the judge call him "indifferent, callous, stubborn, bullheaded." This blunt characterization is so stark, I almost believe it. Hot, sour saliva fills my throat. I swallow hard, but the burn sears my chest, a straight shot to the gut.

Russell Weller was not present when the jurors arrived at the unanimous verdict: guilty on ten felony counts of vehicular manslaughter with gross negligence. "Felony." Meaning Russell Weller is a criminal. "Gross negligence." A reckless disregard for others, so great it appears to be a conscious violation of others' rights and safety. Just shy of being intentionally evil. My gut churns fast and hard as I try to digest the judge's pointed remarks along with the verdict I just read.

A criminal, a violent offender who *wanted* to hurt people. The verdict alone stings too much to digest. Still, I refuse to let myself imagine the relief on Russell Weller's face when he learned he would not serve as much as eighteen years in prison, but was given five years' felony probation plus fines amounting to more than $100,000. Instead, I construct a convulsing, anguished-faced man with his head in his hands, crying and crying and crying—the remorseful, regretful man I need to see.

Lynne's daughter was present in the courtroom with other survivors and families of the dead when the judge delivered the sentence. "I'll never get to see my mom again," she said. "Why should he get to see his family?"

Shamsi's granddaughter: "It's the end of his life. The Weller family members have to deal with their own actions or inactions in not taking away the keys from this man."

Movsha's daughter spoke from hindsight, recognizing that the futures of so many could have turned out for the better: "The City of Santa Monica should bear some responsibility. If the place was adequately protected, more likely it would not have happened, or the extent of injuries would have been minute."

The city, along with Bayside District Corporation, a company that oversees the city's downtown area, did assume responsibility. In 2008, they arrived at a $21 million settlement originating from the forty-two civil suits filed against them, closing the case on one of the worst pedestrian accidents in U.S. history. My share of the settlement was not nearly enough to make up for the lost income I would have earned in the next twenty-five years had I been able to continue working as a critical care nurse. But it helped to close that part of my life and allow me to move on. I was happy to learn that the Farmers' Market acted to improve pedestrian safety. Three years after the settlement, they installed removable dragnets designed from gear used to snare jets on aircraft carriers. Shoppers, vendors, pedestrians, were now better protected—at a modest cost of $219,000. At one point, my medical claims and out-of-pocket expenses alone exceeded that amount. And that doesn't include ongoing treatment for symptoms associated with a TBI and PTSD.

There would be more to come, more pedestrian accidents at open-air events. In 2013, an out-of-control truck killed eight spectators at a Mexican air show. Less than six months later, a twenty-one-year-old drunk driver killed four at a music festival in Austin, Texas. In September 2025, a thirty-seven-year-old woman driving a Honda Odyssey minivan crashed through barricades near an area set up for children's activities at the Kipona Labor Day Festival in Harrisburg, Pennsylvania. Three people were struck, including a six-year-old boy, who was critically injured. The list goes on and on and on.

The escalation of vehicle-ramming attacks from 2014 onward has had another effect. It forced cities large and small to wake-up to the threat of out-of-control cars, and to consider solutions in the form of strategically placed barriers that would allow pedestrians to go about their business, free from the threat of rampaging cars and trucks.

In 2018, the San Luis Obispo Farmers' Market in California fast-tracked their pedestrian safety project; they approved $1.3 million to erect removable steel bollards. The concern for pedestrian safety gained urgency in New York City after a driver, high on PCP, sped three blocks on a Midtown Manhattan sidewalk, followed by the vehicle-ramming attack along the Hudson River. In the wake of these incidents, the city allocated $50 million for better, secure high-risk public spaces. Part of that money was used to install fifteen hundred metal bollards at locations most visited by tourists. Some might gasp at the price tag attached to these barriers, considering the Santa Monica Farmers' Market paid much less for the drag nets. But compare those figures to the collective medical expenses incurred by all sixty-three injured in the Farmers' Market crash, plus the $21 million settlement. Plus medical damages incurred by the injured in New York City, Charlottesville, Toronto, Berlin, Nice.... Now that's sticker-shock.

Bollards and other substantial security barriers are not necessarily imposing or intrusive. They can even beautify the cityscape. When security barriers were needed to protect the entrance to London's Arsenal's Emirates Stadium, designers came up with a creative solution. They placed massive, freestanding concrete letters spelling out the word, ARSENAL, at the main entrance. They serve as a model for how physical barriers can be turned into art. More and more cities have installed large planters, concrete benches, and lampposts to serve the purpose of protection, while adding an aesthetic or functional dimension.

The city of Barcelona has taken the lead and gone beyond erecting bollards to create long-term planning that reimagines the urban future as one in which cars are relegated to the fringes, and pedestrians move freely and safely in an urban landscape that is quieter, greener, and safer. In a big and bold move to stop prioritizing cars—and the attendant noise, pollution, and potential for accidents—Barcelona is constructing so-called "superblocks." Traffic will be restricted to a few, large collector arteries, while secondary streets are being converted into citizen spaces designated for cultural activities, community gatherings, and leisure. This ambitious citywide plan will transform Barcelona, dramatically reducing air pollution and making the city more breathable and livable. It will also save thousands of lives lost to causes ranging from accidents, to heart disease, asthma, and even diabetes.

For Jenna, "It wasn't an accident... he did it on purpose."

For Shamsi, "He was an old man who lost control, and what can we do about that?"

For me, each time I ask myself who is to blame, one word emerges with utter clarity: "Both."

The NTSB's conclusion supports that. They concluded that the crash was due to both pedal error and the lack of an adequate barrier system, which contributed to the severity of the outcome. Both Russell Weller and the City of Santa Monica are to blame. Of course, blame doesn't change the outcome of the accident. But in some inexplicable way, for me, it dulls the sharp fangs of anxiety.

Russell Weller—the man who coldly asked how many people he hit and why we didn't get out of his way—hardly resembles the man portrayed in other news stories as a devoted high-school tutor, organizer of local library book sales, a warm host of holiday gatherings, and a loving uncle who played baseball with his nephew. A man of peace who would never do harm to others. The contrast between the two Russell Weller's is jarringly sharp. I don't know who Russell Weller is, or what to believe. Is he the "stubborn" and "bullheaded" individual the judge characterized? Or the "loving" and "concerned" person his neighbors and long-time pastor described him as?

I decide I can't trust static words on the page, words lacking sound, emotion, pitch. I need to hear Russell Weller's side of the story. Like Lynne's husband, Robby, I need to hear him apologize. "It would have meant a great deal to me and I believe others," he said in the courtroom, "to look him in the eyes and to hear him simply say, 'I'm sorry.'"

What is genuine remorse anyway? When others cause us harm or injury, it can be said that we need them to *do* remorse—shed tears or fall to their knees, for instance. While being held in a detention center in Yokohama, Japan, for hitting and killing a woman, the seventy-four-year-old driver responsible for her death prayed for her survival. When a police officer told him she had died, he collapsed to the floor, weeping as he apologized. That's as real as real gets.

Chapter 51

"I'm not sure it's a good idea," my mother says when I call to tell her I've been thinking about returning to the Farmers' Market. "Being there could re-traumatize you." I'm not surprised by her response. I've always known her to take her worrying seriously, as I do with my fretting over this and that. "You should be careful when you go out," is her advice when she hears news of yet another terrorist attack or hate crime. "Maybe you should hide in the closet" is her go-to humor on a mild worry day. And when I share with her my own anxieties, she'll say, "Don't worry, things will only get worse."

Humor aside, I perseverate about my mother's latest advice as I search JetBlue's website for travel dates to Santa Monica. It's too late; my mother's fear has been passed on to me like DNA. I envision a Melissa walking down Arizona Avenue, arriving at the Farmers' Market, and losing control of her emotions at once: crying, screaming until her throat burns, lashing out blindly, fists and feet striking anything and anyone too close. The overwhelm surges beyond containment. Her composure gives way, and her body buckles, folding in on itself. She hits the ground hard. Sensation drains out of her. She can't feel her heart beating, or hear her own breath. The boundaries of her body blur. She no longer knows if she is real.

I close out the JetBlue website.

John and I discussed my returning to the market weeks before I told my mother, but I hadn't considered how it might affect me until now. "I need to talk to vendors that were there on that day," I had told him. "And I want to see Tina." He understood. "I'll be right there with you."

Returning to the accident site might also be a form of exposure therapy. If I lay myself bare to that potentially anxiety-provoking place, I could master control; I wouldn't shatter into a thousand pieces. I also have this fantastical notion of re-enacting the accident with the ability to change the outcome. But sometimes I visualize the calendar that once hung in my apartment kitchen in Montpelier, and see the month of July displayed, the field of strawberries adorning the top half. Inevitably, I see the sixteenth of July and think, if it were possible to return to that day, to walk the same route to the Farmers' Market, and hold the same peach, would I?

"How come the Jet Blue website is up?" John says later that evening. It's been hours since I thought I X'd out of the page. "Are we going somewhere?" He looks straight at me, as if he hopes I'll say yes.

"I think I'm ready," I say, then pause. "I think I'm ready to go back to Santa Monica."

John claps his hands together. "Yes. I'm in." That same night he finds a flight for February. "All I have to do is hit the confirm button," he says, his hand hovering over the mouse.

The gouge on Shamsi's leg, the port-wine bruise on her forehead, the brace holding her neck in place, flashes across my mind: *she* returned. She found ripe pears.

"Okay, John. Do it."

He jumps up from the chair, bear-hugs me, then steps back and holds my face, his fingers pulsing with warmth. "We're going," he says, pulling me in closer. "We're really going, back to Santa Monica." As he exhales, I inhale. We breathe, together.

I call Tina. "I'll definitely plan to be there with you," she says. "I'll show you the exact route I walked that day."

My next task is to send a letter to Russell Weller. But it takes me another two weeks to get my nerve up to type the first sentence.

"Dear Russell, I've been thinking of you and hope you're doing well." *Too informal?* "Dear Mr. Weller ..." *Too formal?*

Dear Mr. Weller, I was at the Santa Monica Farmers' Market when you hit me, and I ended up in the hospital with severe injuries." *Too Harsh.*

An hour later, maybe two, I get it all on the page:

> Dear Mr. Weller,
> You don't know me, but I wanted to reach out anyway. I sustained severe injuries in the Santa Monica Farmers' Market accident, and still think about that day. I'd like to talk with you, hear from you what you remembered. I'll be in Santa Monica on February 9th and 10th. Please know I mean no harm and look forward to hearing from you.
>
> Warm regards,
> Melissa Cronin

"Is it too direct?" I ask John later that day. "Should I say more? Do you think he'll even read it?"

"It's great. Send it."

I wait two more days to mail the letter. December 7—I hope—will bring me luck, the day Russell Weller turns ninety-two.

Three weeks pass with no response. "If you were Russell Weller, what would you do?" I ask John. He rocks his head side to side against the recliner's backrest, like he does whenever he's contemplating something.

"Well?" I ask.

"I don't know. Sorry." His head rocks faster.

I don't know how I would respond either.

Three. One. Zero. I tap each digit of my cell phone, pulling my hand back after each quick tap, as if I'm tapping the burning end of an incense stick. I'm certain that I'm going completely crazy. But I can't stand waiting any longer. I have to call Russell Weller. I dial all ten digits. A hollow ring sounds, followed by static, then another hollow ring, then more static. My heart knocks against my chest as I anticipate what he might say: "Don't call here again. Leave me alone." A third hollow ring. And then, "The number you have dialed has been disconnected. If you think you dialed the correct number, please hang up and dial again." *Maybe I do have the wrong number. Maybe Russell Weller changed it.* My heart knocks harder. *Maybe he died.*

After receiving no response in the mail, and failing to get through to him by phone, I locate the name of his pastor, and leave a message asking if he would speak with Russell Weller about meeting with me. I never receive a call back. I can't think of any other way for us to connect, other than hiring someone to locate him.

My fingers slip from the keys as I type fast, misspelling private investigator: "Petigateibestigator LA. Pteriistagat. SsamtaMponida." A message spits back, instructing me to try a different spelling. When I do get it right, a long list of names appears. I click on the first one. A webpage pops up with a white background and contact information. No photo. The white expanse puts me in a daze. Before I call, I rehearse what I'll say, annunciating each word loudly, as if I'm delivering a formal speech: "Hello, my name is Melissa Cronin. I'd like to hire you to find George Russell Weller."

"Good afternoon," a male voice answers. "Luis speaking." His tone is clipped, business-like, and peppered with a slight western accent.

"Hi. My name's Melissa, um, Melissa Cronin," I stammer. "I'm trying to locate someone." I don't recognize my own voice. I'm wheezing and try to clear my throat, but can't speak the words in any sensible order. "I think I have the correct address. California. I'm not sure. Do you do that kind of thing?"

"Are you looking for a family member?" he asks.

"No. I'm—I'm trying to find someone. A man. He's not a family member. George Russell Weller." I speak his entire name slowly and precisely. "There was an accident," I say. "He drove through the Santa Monica Farmers' Market. I need to find him, because ... I just need to find him."

The line goes quiet. I wonder if Luis has hung up.

He coughs. "Yes, I remember that accident," he says, his clipped business tone now a drawl. "One of my employees, Gloria, was there." His voice is unsteady. "She was killed."

I think I'm going to pass out. Is this some weird, cosmic connection? Or plain randomness? "I'm so sorry," I say. "I called you because your name was the first one to come up in my search. I swear. I had no idea you knew her."

Luis continues speaking about Gloria, as if he hasn't in a long time and needs to. Without stopping for a breath, the words spill out of him. "She worked for me for several years, she moved here from Mexico, she had kids, a husband." He stops, breathes. "Her body was trapped under the car. They couldn't even have an open casket. Why do you want to find him?"

"I don't mean to cause any harm. I'll be in Santa Monica soon and want to meet him. He hasn't responded to a letter I sent him. He doesn't answer the phone."

"Sorry," Luis says, "but I don't think showing up at Russell Weller's home is the right thing to do."

Wait a minute? I think. Whose side is he on? Gloria was killed. Why wouldn't he want to know what Russell Weller has to say? "It could be considered harassment," he cautions, "or trespassing, if you show up at his house. If you insist on going, you should hire a police escort." *Harassment. Trespassing. Police.* Now I feel like some kind of evil secret agent. Cold. Cruel. Calculating.

Have I crossed the line, from the woman who once so willingly caved in to others, to a woman who now refuses to listen? I don't know how to respond to Luis, other than to apologize for bothering him, and to thank him for his time.

With the image of Gloria trapped under the car, I search Google for her photo. Among other photos of those who were killed in the accident, Gloria's gaze meets mine: black-olive eyes framed by high cheekbones. She looks healthy, energetic, with her sun-glazed complexion and full lips. Beneath her photo, in unmistakable traditional font, is her age. Thirty-five. Gloria, who rode the bus seventeen miles to the Farmers' Market to buy wholesome produce for her family, then stepped off, but never got back on. Instead, her family brought her back to Oaxaca, where they buried her in her native soil.

If I did cross the line, I can't step back to the other side now. I email the attorney who represented me in the civil case against the City of Santa Monica:

> Hi Mr. Archer. I'm traveling to Santa Monica in a few days to visit the Farmers' Market. I sent a letter to Russell Weller in December asking to meet with him, but didn't hear back. I've heard he's homebound with twenty-four-hour nursing care. Do you know any more about his condition?

Two hours pass before Mr. Archer responds: "I recall from the last time I saw Russell Weller he was very old and frail. He sometimes appeared lucid. I'm sure his condition has deteriorated and his frailty has increased."

My eyes water from staring too long at the word "frail." I close the laptop, then open it again to read the email a second time, as if that could magically change Mr. Archer's response: "Russell Weller is doing well. He's stronger than you'd expect." Of course, the response is the same, and I close the lid, the latch clicking into place. I putter around the living room, not knowing what to do with myself, stop at the sliding glass door, and slide back the curtain. A titanium corona surrounds the full moon. I slide the shade closed. Later, I pull it back open. I want to see the circle of light, but it has retreated into the inkblot sky.

Chapter 52

As John and I walk into the candlelit restaurant on Fifth Street and Santa Monica Avenue, I squint at the tall slender man standing by a table ten feet away. That can't be him, I think, surprised by Brett's six-foot frame as I approach him. "Really, you're the same Brett I met six and a half years ago?" I ask.

"Yes," Tina says, standing next to her son. "He's still the same Brett you met when I brought him to visit you at Cedars. Caring, loving, interested."

"I'll be eighteen in a few days," Brett says. His baritone voice strikes me as impossible. How did it change so fast? How did he get to be so big, when it didn't seem too long ago that he was only four feet tall?

Tina appears short next to her son, much shorter than I remember from when she visited me at Cedars. All of my memories from then are imprinted from the perspective of my wheelchair. And her hair is still long and the same light brown.

She hugs me tight, holding me with the same flower garden scent I remember from her visit at Cedars. "I've heard so much about you, John. It's great to finally meet you." She hugs him tight, too, as if she's known him for years.

"So, Melissa, are you ready for tomorrow?" Tina asks, settling into a chair next to Brett.

"I suppose so. I'm glad you can come with us."

"Of course. I cleared my calendar for the entire day."

I drop into the chair next to John. *Fifteen.* The number of hours until we'll be back at the market.

As we sit, Tina opens her memory chest, releasing pent-up worry dust. "I don't know if I already told you this, but it took me two days to find you at the hospital. I needed to find you, to make sure you were okay. I called all the hospitals in the area." She holds her fist to her ear, shaking it, as though making an urgent call, begging the person on the other end to please find me.

"I had no idea it took you so long," I say, sinking into that apologetic place I often find myself in when there's nothing at all to be sorry about. If I knew where I was going when the rescue workers flew off with me in the helicopter, I could have told Tina where to find me. How scared and worried she must have been. I reach for the arm of my chair, grounding myself against the solid surface.

"I had this dream," Brett says. "It was a few days after the accident. A car drove through a bunch of people, but no one was hurt. I haven't forgotten that dream." Brett wasn't at the market that day, yet he saw and heard it on television: downed vendor poles and canopies, smashed produce, covered bodies, sirens and screams. He sits taller, draws a breath. "The blood must have been everywhere, because when you came home, Mom, it was all over your blouse." His voice cracks, as if he's a preadolescent boy again.

I gulp some water, cool my anxiety with a melting ice cube.

What exactly did Tina tell her eleven-year-old son? That there was an accident, but not to worry? I didn't ask, because I wasn't sure what I'd do if I had children.

"I headed right for the bathtub," Tina says.

"That's right," Brett agrees. "Dad asked me not to disturb you while you soaked in the tub." He leans into his mother and rubs her back.

"Melissa, you might not remember this," Tina says, "but the rescue workers labeled each victim with a tag." Using her fingers to count, she names each one. "Green. Red. Black."

"Black?" I say. "I thought there was only green, for stable, and red, for urgent. But black?"

Tina and Brett respond in unison. "Black for dead."

Black. Dead. Those two words wallop me voiceless.

John takes my hand.

Tina leans forward, her hands folded on the table. "Once the rescue workers carried you to the helicopter, one of them said, 'If you didn't stay with her, she would've died, right there, on the pavement.'"

I shudder, squeezing John's hand. He squeezes back, his hand warm, mine cold. He doesn't have to repeat the promise he made to me on our second date: "I'm going to work hard to make sure you're safe."

A part of me thinks I should have listened to my mother. Returning will shake me upside down; it will take considerable muscle to keep me upright. I could have asked Tina not to share the details, but I need to know, as gruesome as they are. And it's obvious she needs to talk, to resurrect the details. I remember our phone conversation from six years ago. I had asked Tina if she had spoken with anyone about the horror she witnessed. "I'm doing well," she said. "I'm fine." And that was that.

As the server sets down our dinner plates, garlic and Dijon distracts me from the black tags. I bite into a forkful of salmon. It falls apart in my mouth. Mild and creamy. *I can do this.*

"I knew my employees would worry about me," Tina continues. "I had to go back to work. But I could see the body on the hood of the car from my office window."

I bite down hard on my cheek. Salt. Blood.

How could Tina not have PTSD? Soon after I returned to Vermont, I wrote in my letter to the Santa Monica Chamber of Commerce that "bystanders had to bear witness to such an unexpected massacre," implying they must have suffered emotional harm. At the time, I had yet to undergo PTSD treatment and didn't have a name for the bystanders' suffering. But all these years later, after EMDR, after reading books and research articles and blogs about trauma, I know that not only those who suffer direct injury from a tragedy but witnesses of such trauma are at risk of developing PTSD, too.

"The body was there all afternoon while the police investigated the scene," she says.

I drop my fork onto the plate, the tines clanking against ceramic. I didn't see or hear what Tina saw: the speeding Buick, the downed vendor stands, pedestrians lying next to me, their limbs crushed and twisted.

Chapter 53

The following morning, John and I walk the few blocks from our hotel to Tina's office. The sun hazes over us like yellow wax. Heat rises from the sidewalk, wrapping around my bare legs. Homeless men crouch against buildings, holding flimsy cardboard signs: "Out of work. Anything will do. God bless." Something tugs at me from inside. I remember the man I passed when walking to the market six and a half years ago, the empty amber bottle next to him, the tattered box he slept behind. I remember how thirsty and hungry I was; so was he. Another tug: fifty-five-year-old Leroy Lattier.

While researching the stories of those who died, I learned Leroy was homeless after moving from Louisiana to Santa Monica in search of expert treatment for his diabetes. In an unfamiliar city, he took any job he could find. On that July day, working with the Farmers' Market clean-up crew, he held himself up on crutches as he swiped his broom along Arizona Avenue, brushing wind-blown napkins, fruit pits, and corn silk into a dustpan. The moment he was struck by the Buick, he went airborne, his crutches collapsing beneath him.

"This must be it," John says, as we approach Tina's office building. He opens the heavy door to the entrance, and I step over the threshold onto a white-tiled floor, cool air falling on my neck and shoulders.

A receptionist stands up from behind a counter and walks over to us, her chiffon skirt swishing. "You must be Melissa and John," she says. "Tina's expecting you. I'll let her know you're here." She shakes my hand, her fingers like silk against my wintered palm.

The elevator doors shush open, and Tina steps out, ready for the walk to the market in her black jeans and a gray t-shirt. She waves for us to step into the elevator. "I want to show you my office first." And the doors shush closed.

Her carpeted office is furnished with a glass coffee table in front of a leather sofa. Opposite the table and sofa is a desk the color of roasted chestnut. "That's so I can watch the basketball and football games," she says, pointing to the flat-screen television on the wall behind the couch. Framed posters of band logos—Cream, Taj Mahal, Joan Baez and Bob Dylan, Country Joe and the Fish—line the overhang to the left of her desk. A limited-edition poster of The Grateful Dead in Egypt hangs on the wall next to the television. Most of the posters are from concerts Tina went to in the sixties and seventies. I know she works as a financial advisor for people in the entertainment industry, but I don't understand why she chose to work with musicians. "You never told me about your interest in music," I say.

"These define the foundation of my youth," she explains, pointing to the posters. "Without this soundtrack of my life, I'd be a very different person, or perhaps not here at all."

I linger in front of the posters for a few minutes, then walk to the glass doors leading to the patio overlooking Wilshire Boulevard, where she now stands talking with John. Their voices sound far away, as if they're in another room. I stare at my ghostly reflection in the glass, wondering what Tina meant by "not here at all." If music were not in the soundtrack of her life, she might not have been at the Farmers' Market on that July day. She would not have knelt by my side and poured cold water down my back, yelled out for the firefighter to tell him I was not okay, that I needed immediate medical attention. I would have died, right there, on the pavement. Wearing the wrong color tag on my toe.

"Let's go," I tell John, interrupting his conversation with Tina. I step away from the glass, an irregular circle of condensation like a misshapen face left behind from my breath.

The three of us walk from Fourth Street to Wilshire Boulevard, toward the Third Street Promenade less than a mile away. As we make our way down the promenade, I count each step, trying to avoid the cracks out of respect for my worrying mother. A man calls out, "Let Christ, our Lord, lead the way." A street performer plays the djembe, his hands percussing its rawhide with urgency, as if he has something he needs to say, but I can't figure out the rhythm. I hear the drummer and the preacher shouting the same thing: *Stop before it's too late! Do not take one more step farther toward the market!*

At the intersection of the promenade and Arizona Avenue, Tina stops. She pirouettes like a ballerina, looks up at the sky, as if searching for a lost balloon. "Right here, I went to step off of this curb. Then I saw a car racing toward me from the direction of Fourth Street." She points. "It sped so close my hair blew in my face." A gentle wind blows my own hair. She points to the long row of vendors. "Then I heard what sounded like forks banging together. I thought it was music, like cymbals, then realized those clanging sounds were the posts crashing to the ground as the car hit them." It dawns on me. The *pop* I heard, the *pop* I thought was a gunshot, was the Buick striking a vendor post. I stick my fingers in my ears. *Bzzzz*, like an electric current moving through high-tension wires.

Tina sweeps her hand from right to left, showing us how the Buick moved straight through one side of the market, bringing the posts down. "He was staring directly ahead," she says, "in panic, in fear." *Boom, boom, boom.* I jump back into John's solid arms.

We turn right, walk past a large, bright-orange Road Closed Ahead sign, past two police cars blocking the market's entrance. No plastic A-frame barriers. There must be a hundred tables, two rows lining each side of Arizona Avenue. Canopies—blue, white, green—flap in the offshore breeze. John holds my hand as we head toward Second Street, passing slender asparagus bunches, spinach bouquets, sweet Vidalia onions. Older people shuffle along, some using walkers, others with canes. *What did Russell Weller say to the police about losing his cane? "I lose it a couple times a week."* The hairs on my arms and neck stand up stiff. We weave past a mother pushing a carriage with a toddler. I look back at it, envisioning its intact wheels and handlebars as the twisted, lone stroller I read about in a newspaper article. Who sat in that stroller? Brandon? Cindy? I try to enjoy the guy strumming folk music on his guitar, but it isn't loud enough to silence the *crunch* of aluminum in my head.

The three of us stop at a vendor selling kale. "Excuse me, this is Melissa," Tina says, gesturing for me to step closer toward him. "She was injured here, in the accident."

He drops a head of kale he's holding, scattering moist soil along the table. A thirty-something-year-old, he gives me a zealous handshake. He smells like freshly cut grass. "I was here that day," he says. "One of my workers had just handed me a watermelon." He pantomimes placing it into a phantom truck bed behind him, his hands mostly muscle and tendon. "Then I set the watermelon down, and heard the posts crashing to the ground." I step back, away from the posts holding up the canopy, and nearly trip over my own feet, but John catches me. "I saw bodies flying," he says, moving his hand above his head in a long arc. "I ran after the car. I helped lift it up off a body." He squats, holding his hands out, his face flushing, beads of sweat forming on his nose as he re-enacts the moment when he used all his effort to lift the car. *Gloria. She was trapped . . . couldn't even have an open casket.* I bite the tender part of my cheek I bit the evening before, when Tina told me about the body she saw from her office window. Now I don't need to be told if the body beneath the car was male or female. It must have been Gloria. The vendor sees me shaking and wraps his arms around me, his full-bodied hold tells me they are the same strong arms that tried to save Gloria. I hold onto him—to the smell of watermelon and grass.

We cross the street, toward a fruit stand on the other side of Arizona Avenue. Tina introduces me to another vendor, someone she knows from shopping at the market. He stares at me with his mouth wide open when I tell him I was injured. "There's so much I still remember," he starts. "The car dragged a body down the road." The body *thumps* and *thumps*, *thumps* again, beneath my skull. He swings his arm to the side, in the direction the Buick traveled, telling us how Russell Weller sped for two-and-a-half blocks before he stopped, a body beneath his car. I lean into John. The *lub-dub* in my chest slows.

"I had to jump out of the way," he says. "The car was that close to me." He hops back, off the street and onto the sidewalk. John and I flinch and take a step backward.

Neither of the vendors mention the body on the hood of the Buick, the same body Tina saw from her office window. I still don't understand how she could have seen it from her office. I dig my nails deep into my arms.

While the vendor helps a customer, and Tina picks out some oranges, I whisper to John, "What about the other body, the one Tina said she saw from her office?"

He lays his hand on my shoulder, looks at me with a crooked grin. "Melissa, she saw it in her mind. It was burned in. She didn't actually see the body from her office." Now I get it, what she meant about seeing the body from her window. It is her private window, one which only she can see through. I shield my eyes with my hand, and block my private view of the covered body with the sandals sticking out, the rescue worker with his head hanging low. And the black tags.

The vendor apologizes for making us wait and picks up where he left off. "The car swerved."

"What?" I ask, remembering reporters saying Russell Weller sped straight ahead, his hands in the ten-and-two position.

"It swerved," he repeats, "the car."

I step farther away from the street, closer to the oranges. *Why didn't people get out of my way? Yes, that's what Russell Weller said.* I feel the same sting to the face I felt when reading that reaction from him in news articles. A pressure pushes against my sternum with such force I want to scream it out of me: "If we knew which goddam direction you were about to swerve, maybe we could get out of your way."

As I start walking with Tina and John toward another vendor, a childlike voice from behind me catches my attention. A slight woman wearing an ankle-length floral skirt stands a few inches away, her blue eyes staring at me. Her name is Sonia. She says she knows one of the vendors I just spoke with, and that he pointed me out in the crowd. "I was here on that day, too," she says. She touches her thigh, showing me where muscle tissue had been damaged. "My friends threw me out of the way when they saw the car coming." Sonia leaps onto the grass on the other side of the sidewalk, as if she expects the Buick to charge toward her at any moment.

"I remember it all," she says. "I don't want to forget."

Do I want to remember?

Tina guides John and me to another fruit stand. "Right here," she says, pointing to the ground beneath her. This is where I found you." The three of us stand close together. There's too much noise: squawking seagulls, intersecting voices, a police siren sounding in the distance. A haphazard spread of tangerines covers the table—peaches are not in season. I look at the ground where I once lay. I step back, as if I just stepped on someone's grave, bend down, and touch the black strip of hardened tar. Quickly, I withdraw my hand from the hot strip. What used to be under there? Blood? Glass? Skin? Who else once lay near that spot? Shamsi, Sandra, Ilona? So many people now walk over it.

I close my eyes, pretend I am lying on that blackened patch, looking up at the pulsing blue sky, and whisper to myself, "The ground will hold me in its warmth. I am alive and safe and unafraid."

Chapter 54

John drives through the palm-treed neighborhoods of Santa Monica with me next to him in the passenger seat, my hands sweating, my heart beating through my ribs. We're on our way to Russell Weller's house. But first, we decide to stop at a nearby grocery store and cafe so I can get some soothing tea and reevaluate, as I have done again and again over the past few months, whether showing up at his house is the right thing to do.

Among the store's display of hibiscus, tiger lilies, and orchids, my eyes land on a lone sweetheart rose plant. I pick it up. The deep red petals smell like clean lake water. "John, I want to bring this to Russell Weller's." It's Valentine's Day, and I can't think of a better time to offer a gesture of goodwill.

As we make our way through the produce section, greens, yellows, and oranges come at me in a blur. The sudden rumble of a blender scares the shit out of me. I stop, look around, trying to figure out which way to walk. John recognizes my dazed stare and reaches for my hand. "Hon, the tea's over here."

We've been married for five and a half years, and John knows me well. He knows when I'm experiencing brain fog, and has become used to my heightened startle response and hypervigilance. John holds my hand a lot, not only in stores, but when crossing the street. John has become my compass, helping me find my way along the sharp turns of unfamiliar and sometimes familiar roads. But because he understands that I also need space and time to test my ability to take certain risks, to figure out for myself which routes are safe to walk along, he knows when to gently let go of my hand, and when to reach for it again.

One block, two blocks, left on Twenty-Fifth Street. My feet press hard against the floor mats of the car. I have no idea what kind of man I will meet. Of course, I'm keeping my fingers crossed, hoping to meet a welcoming man. But the Russell Weller who has a reputation for being gentle might not be the Russell Weller I will meet at all. He's now ninety-three, and from what I read in news articles, he is ill and needs twenty-four-hour nursing care. If he can't make it to the door, maybe someone else will answer. What if they refuse to let me in and slam the door in my face? What then? Before John and I left for California, friends asked, "Have you thought about what you'll do if he or his family get angry with you for showing up?" No, I still have not.

Gallant brick homes with rolled-out lawns and smoothly paved driveways line the neighborhood. "John, do you think it's that one?" I point at a three-story house with an arched entryway surrounded by topiary bushes.

"No, this is it," he says, as he edges the car up to the curb, and stops in front of a beige, one-level ranch. The engine hisses. My heart beats in stutters. No life seems to exist in or around the house: vacant driveway, closed windows, drawn shades. But the lawn is green and well-manicured; someone must be taking care of it, maybe Russell Weller's nephew or a neighbor. A little girl is playing in the yard across the street, and I wonder if her family knows Russell Weller, if it's a better idea to talk with them first. Maybe they'll introduce me to him, help make my uninvited appearance a little less awkward.

No, I have to do this on my own. I hold my breath; I've forgotten how to exhale. I think about Russell Weller's darkened living room behind closed shades. If he's dozing in a recliner or hospital bed, my knock will startle him awake. What if he sees me from behind the shade? What if he calls the police? What if his niece is there and screams at me, "Get off our property!" What will I do then? Run off? Plead with her to let me meet her uncle? "I understand he's ill, but please, let me speak with him."

Though I believe he never intended any harm, I need to hear his perspective about what happened on that July day six and a half years ago. I need to know—from him—if he has any regrets at all about driving to the post office, if he wishes he had listened to his wife instead and waited for the postman to pick up the letter for his niece. Has the accident changed him? How? It has certainly changed me.

"Go ahead," John says. "You can do it." Trembling, I open the car door and step onto the sidewalk in front of the house. I feel a squeezing sensation in my chest, as if my heart is compressing in on itself. With each squeeze, I clasp my hands tighter around the miniature rose plant I bought that morning. *It's Valentine's Day. What could possibly go wrong?* I walk ahead, and pause at the head of the driveway to take a deep breath. My heart keeps squeezing, pounding, blood banging through me. I grip the plant tighter, as if I can transfer all my anxiety into the soil and bury it there. *Stay with it, Melissa. Don't you fucking turn back now.*

I step over the winding crack at the edge of the driveway, and as though someone might hear my footsteps, I tiptoe the twenty feet toward the stone walkway leading to the front steps. As my foot lands on the second step, a stone wiggles loose, detonating a blast of adrenaline. I face the door. The doorbell is an arm's reach away. I see a flash of red from my peripheral vision, and turn my head left. Red capitalized letters are pasted across a black mailbox. NO SOLICITORS hits me in the eye like an assault. I stumble back, away from the bright burning caution. The petals quivering under the aftershocks of my shiver, I bend down, set the plant in front of the door, then stand up and hurry back toward the car, my heart skipping, pounding harder, faster with each step. I jerk open the car door, and slump down into the seat.

"You did it," John says.

I watch Russell Weller's house, my eyes looping from the sun-scorched shutters to the faded siding to the drawn shades, back to the front stoop with the rose plant. Did he receive the letter I had sent him in the fall? If so, maybe he'll assume it's me who brought the plant. Or maybe I should have left a note. Maybe I should have ignored the red caution and knocked on the door, taken the chance.

"Do you think you can let it go now?" John asks.

I claw my fingernails into my arms, trying to release the disappointment and anger building up in me like a toxin.

"I don't think so."

How can I let it go? As my friend said when he called me at Cedars six and a half years ago, I'll never be the same again. Sandra, Ilona, Jenna, Bartley, and so many others, including Russell Weller, will never be the same again. But he still has the freedom to make choices. He can choose to remain in hiding, his only communication with the outside world a glaring-red No Solicitors sign, while Brandon, Cindy, Gloria, Diana, Lynne, Theresa, Kevin, Leroy, Molok, and Movsha have lost the opportunity to choose at all. They are dead; Russell Weller is still alive. And so am I, fully alive—happily married, playing my fiddle, chasing after leaves, and continuing to rebuild my brain.

I'll often go for a walk, in search of a quiet place to sit. On my walk, I always tread along the part of the sidewalk farthest from the road. I'll look left, right, left, and right again before crossing the street. Sometimes the walk takes longer than I expected, but that doesn't matter. I'll keep going, hoping I'll eventually find my way to that tranquil, uninterrupted place.

Chapter 55

On December 9, 2010, two days after his ninety-fourth birthday, Russell Weller dies. I cry hard when I learn of his death. I cry because I've been hoping for a long time now that I might have the chance to meet him, even if I've known all along how far-fetched that hope is, especially after coming face to face with the No Solicitors sign. His pastor, whom I reached out to two weeks before returning to the market, might have called to say Russell Weller wanted to meet with me after all. Russell Weller himself might have called me. I cry because I'm angry with myself for backing away from the No Solicitors sign, for not pressing the doorbell on that Valentine's Day. Instead, I let both doubt and fear stalk me like twin predators. I cry because now I must let go of my need to meet him; his death has made it certain that will never happen. But I don't know how to let go. Russell Weller, who quite literally barged into my life seven years ago, has taken up residence in my mind. His face, his imagined voice has lived in my head, day after day, all these years. I still need to hear from him, to hear him express remorse, to see for myself that he, too, has felt the accumulated pain, grief, and loss he caused, that he has confronted the horror of what he has done. I also need to know, exactly, how it happened from his point of view. The concept of pedal error, unintentionally stepping on the gas pedal instead of the brake, seems like a neat and reductive explanation for what took place. What was going through Russell Weller's head as he sped up to sixty miles an hour over the course of twenty seconds and two-and-a-half blocks, as people ran screaming and bodies bounced off the hood of his car?

Will I ever know?

A few months after Russell Weller's death, during a conversation with a friend about the Farmers' Market crash, he asks how his death affected me. "I still can't believe I was standing right there," I say, "on his doorstep, and walked away."

"There must be a recording of him talking to the police," he says. "I'm sure you could get a copy."

I give myself a whap to the forehead. "Why didn't I think of that?" I feel like a jump-started battery. A new energy fills me from my eyeballs to my pinky toes.

First thing the next morning, I call the Los Angeles courts, the Los Angeles district attorney's office, court clerks, the head deputy of the Santa Monica police, anyone who might know where and how to get the recording. I'm sure it has to be on file somewhere.

"Yes," the head deputy says, when he returns my call that same day. "A copy of the video will be in the mail to you tomorrow."

A video. My heartbeat skips all over the place. This is it, finally, my chance to see and hear Russell Weller tell his story of what happened that day.

A week later, the video arrives, the envelope labeled "fragile." Carefully, I peel back the seal, and there it is, with a white sticker affixed to the DVD: "SMPD Interview of George Russell Weller, July 16, 2003."

My hands shaking, I slide the disc into the DVD player, and sit cross-legged on the carpet, inches from the television. Grey, black, and white static wash across the screen. A digital clock then starts its count in the upper right-hand corner: *15:10, 15:11, 15:12.* The police tape of the interview begins at 3:10 p.m., one hour and twenty-three minutes after Russell Weller sped down Arizona Avenue, collapsing fruit stands and sending umbrellas and people flying.

The static clears, bringing into focus a bare, white-walled square room, furnished with only a long wooden table and three vinyl chairs. My eyes burn wide open with anticipation. The digital timer continues its agonizingly slow scroll for four knuckle-cracking minutes. Then Russell Weller enters the room. His presence freezes me in place. All I can feel is my pulse pushing against my inner ear. His physical appearance is exactly what I remembered from news articles, exactly what I imagined him to be: an aging man of medium stature, white-haired, white-mustached, bespectacled, hunched-over, shuffling slowly with a cane. He sits down in a corner of the room, faces the camera, and starts tapping his cane against the concrete floor, pausing to pick at what appears to be bruises on his arm. He scans all four walls, sets his gaze on the peeling ceiling. "Can you imagine?" he whispers.

My hand moves, rises toward my chest, landing instinctively on the area over my heart. I hold it there, waiting—waiting with Russell Weller in that empty, cold room. Alone. He picks at his arm, picks at his cuticles. His eyes scan the room, floor to ceiling, ceiling to floor. His anxiety claws at my stomach.

A baby-faced investigator, wearing a black suit jacket, comes into the room. "I appreciate you volunteering to come down here," he says. "You're not under arrest, or in trouble."

"I'm in trouble with my heart and soul," Russell Weller says. "That you can't fix."

His voice, wavering and weak, stops my breath. *This is it.* I scoot closer to the television.

I'm crying, and I hope Russell Weller will cry too. I need him to cry, then I'll be convinced he's in trouble with his heart and soul. But he does not shed a single tear. I let him off the hook. There's still time. Two hours and fourteen minutes.

The baby-faced investigator leaves, returning every five or ten minutes to tell Russell Weller supervisors will be there soon to talk with him. During those quiet moments, alone again, he sips water from a Dixie cup the investigator gave him. Between sips, he fidgets with his belt buckle, taps his fingernails on the table, mumbles to himself, does everything it takes to hold his shit together.

The clock reads 16:11, an hour after he and I are left waiting. A fit woman with shoulder-length blonde hair, and wearing a sleeveless black top, walks into the room. A heavyset man with thinning dark hair, dressed casually in a white, short-sleeved shirt and jeans, follows behind.

They introduce themselves—Virginia and Eddie—and shake Russell Weller's hand. "Have a seat," he says, smiling, and points to the two chairs opposite him.

Even if this is proof of his reputation as a neighborly man, it strikes me as odd that Russell Weller is playing host to two strangers who are about to do just as he offered: take opposite sides to him.

It strikes me as odd that he smiles.

Virginia pulls her chair closer to Russell Weller. "Thank you for coming in," she says.

"What's my alternative?" he asks. "It happened, and we need to find out how."

My body hardens. *It? Find out how?* As if someone, or something, other than himself is to blame. As if he wasn't the one behind the wheel, with his foot on the accelerator.

"We're really in the dark," Eddie says. "So, we need to know how it happened."

"Me, too," I say, speaking to Eddie's bald spot.

First, he wants to know what Russell Weller's day was like before the accident.

"I had a normal night's rest," he says. "Then got up around 7:30, took a look at the newspaper, showered, figured out what we needed from the store, which didn't amount to diddly. And I went out to get them, then came home."

"What happened next?" Eddie asks, his pen poised on a pad of paper.

"I finished a letter to my niece, who was getting married. And when I finished it, my wife said, 'Are you going to put it out for Ernie?' And I did something I'll remember the rest of my life. I said, 'No. I think I'll take it to the post office to make sure it gets there.'" He tosses his hands up in the air. "If I had only given it to Ernie and gone back in and sat on the couch and minded my own damn business."

"Yes!" I shout, my legs pressing into the carpet. "If only you had given up your car keys before that."

"So, I came down to the post office, threw the letter in the hand drop." Russell Weller raises his arm, traces the wall beside him with his pointer finger, mapping the direction he had driven when he left the post office. "I came down Fifth Street, leaving the post office, to the corner of Arizona. I turned right and saw the Farmers' Market. And as I turned right, I can't give any reason why, but the automobile was accelerating." He's nodding with confusion, his arms limp on his lap.

"How could you not know why the car was accelerating?" I ask out loud, as if the television's speaker is a two-way radio. "How could you not see that it was *you* who made the car accelerate, not see that it was *your* foot on the gas pedal. That it was *you* who made the car speed at sixty miles an hour?" I wonder what Eddie and Virginia are thinking as they sit there with their backs to me, silent, Virginia with her legs crossed, leaning forward, waiting for more.

"I have no idea how many people I hit or how many people I hurt," Russell Weller says. "I'm deeply, deeply sorry for the pain everyone went through. And it was my fault."

He speaks so quietly I can't be sure if I hear what I think I hear. I pause the video, rewind it, shift close to the television, close enough that I can taste static. Over and over, I play it. "I'm deeply, deeply sorry... it was my fault."

I continue watching, listening. If he can't cry, I need some other demonstrable proof of his regret.

"In the course of that one block, when I knocked over those stands, hit those people, and finally came to a rest, I thought, 'My God, what have I done?'"

"I." Good. Please, no more "it."

For the next ten minutes, Russell Weller answers questions about his car and his health. Yes, he brought his Buick in for regular maintenance. Yes, his car had been previously damaged when a car backed into his two years earlier. Yes, I want to grab him by the throat when he laughs out loud and says, "In fact, the car ran a little better after that, but I didn't tell anyone."

“So, you have no problem feeling the gas pedal or the brake?” Eddie asks.

“No,” Russell Weller says, his voice as strong and confident as a politician’s.

“Sir, how long have you been retired?”

“Twenty-two years.” Russell Weller sits up a little taller—smiling.

“What did you do for work?”

“I was a food broker. The company sold out. They couldn’t do it without me.” Another smile.

I reach for the remote next to me, about to hit the exit button. I want so much to turn off his smile. I don’t deserve this. But I grit my teeth, and tell myself to hold tight. *It can’t get any worse.*

“We had a thing that happened,” Russell Weller says, referencing his work. “Incidentally, to get off the subject of today, and I’d like to get off that subject.”

That’s when I pause the video and scream, “You have to be kidding me? You’re sitting there, alive, with not a single scratch, while I was unconscious, in the operating room, bleeding. People died because of you!”

He already crushed me with his Buick. Now he’s at it again, inflicting more damage, wearing me down, breaking to smithereens my inclination to forgive. I’m not sure I can watch any more. And yet I do.

“I want to go back to the post-office,” Eddie says, to clarify it was a curbside mailbox Russell Weller pulled up to when he mailed the letter. “Did you keep your foot on the brake? Or did you put the car in park?”

“I put it in park.”

“As you proceeded, about to make a right turn, what’s the next thing you remember?”

“The next thing I knew, the car was accelerating, and I have no reason to know why.”

“Was your foot on the accelerator?”

“I don’t know. If my foot was on the accelerator, I never, never drive at the speed that thing was accelerating.” Russell Weller places his hand over his chest. “I went through that place, and God help those poor people who were there. Do you have any feedback about what happened?”

“What happened?” I yell at him, unable to wrap my head around such an absurd question. “You were there. You tell us what happened.” His eyes are hollow, his face sagging. He has no idea. No idea that I was barely conscious, still bleeding at that time. No idea that Brandon was bleeding from his ears, that surgeons were pumping blood into Kevin, and that Bartley was in critical condition with a brain injury.

"A little bit," is all Virginia has to say about what she knows, then launches into her own line of questioning. "If you're a camera looking down on to Arizona, do you remember any cars in front of you?" She gestures with her hands as if they're the camera.

"I wished to God I did know. That's the whole market there, from Second to Fourth."

Virginia leans in closer to Russell Weller. "Before you hit Fourth Street, do you remember any cars in front of you?"

"I went around Fourth Street, just around the corner –"

"That's from Fifth Street on to Arizona," Virginia interrupts.

"I went around that corner."

Again, Virginia interrupts, this time using her hands to enact a steering wheel. "Okay, now you're driving down Arizona and you're looking at the Farmers' Market –"

"And the next thing you know I'm going faster than hell."

"Do you remember any cars before you?" Virginia asks again, her hands now fisted in front of her.

"I couldn't get there. I was all but between the Farmers' Market and eternity."

"What is that supposed to mean?" I ask an answerless Russell Weller sitting slack-jawed with a vacant stare.

"I want to understand," Eddie says. "It's your recollection there were no other vehicles between you and the Farmers' Market? Is that correct?"

Russell Weller nods. As much as they try, neither Eddie nor Virginia can yank the answer they seem to want from this utterly unaware and obtuse man.

"As you're approaching the Farmers' Market, and you're driving, do you remember seeing what was in front of you?" Virginia asks, her hands clenched around an imaginary steering wheel. "Could you see the barricades?"

"I could see those barricades."

"What happened with those barricades?"

"That's what I hit. And I took my foot off the brake and tried to find out if I took it off the accelerator. From there on in, all I can remember is *bang, bang, bang.*" His hand slaps the air. Left to right. Right to left.

I fold forward, bury my head between my crossed legs.

"Something hit my windshield and near shattered it."

My head flings up straight, and my eyes focus squarely on Russell Weller's poker face.

"Do you know what it was that hit your windshield?" Virginia asks, referring to the bodies that bounced off the hood of the Buick Le Sabre as it barreled through the crowd of shoppers.

"I have no idea."

The dead, all ten names, land in my head with a slam.

16:40. Less than an hour left. Hang in there, Melissa.

"My feeling is that it accelerated on the turn, and never went back to normal acceleration."

I scoot back from the television, gut punched by another "it." Anger rips through me like a firestorm. I sob and shout at Russell Weller's wooden expression and maddeningly evasive choice of words. "What happened to 'It was my fault'? Why do you keep blaming the car? What the fuck is wrong with you?"

"Do you recall what finally made you stop?" Virginia asks.

Russell Weller throws his hands up. "I guess... I don't know. Maybe I rammed it into park?"

I don't believe him. How can he not know? His casual tone and quick stab at a guess sound much like a cop-out, as if he's turning his head the other way, away from the much larger and viscerally unforgettable reality. The woman trapped beneath the car.

I think I'll rip in two when Eddie asks Russell Weller the last time he renewed his driver's license, and he says, "I lucked out. I passed on the written test high enough where they didn't ask me to drive." My anger flares as I remember the day years ago, when I was listening to the NPR broadcast about older drivers, and Joe Grotsky was saying how lucky he was that he'd be able to keep his license, even though he didn't do well on the written part. I want to grab Russell Weller by the shoulders, turn him upside down, and hear him say again, "I'm deeply, deeply sorry." There isn't enough water nearby to put out the fire consuming me. I want to extinguish it. I don't like the feeling, the boiling over of anger, how close I feel to losing all control over my emotions. I breathe my way through the fire.

"Do I post a bond?" Russell Weller asks. "Do I go to jail?" His voice quiets. "God knows you're going to hear from the people who were injured." Then the *tap, tap, tapping* of his cane as he says, "Would I believe me?" referring to whether the accident was his fault. "I'm not sure I could say yes. Did I step on the accelerator?" He looks at Eddie. "But I would have stepped off it."

The tip of his cane comes down hard. "I have a feeling I re-accelerated three or four times."

"It was the vehicle itself?" Virginia asks.

"It seemed to me it was the vehicle itself responding, because I sure as hell didn't have control over it. I was trying my best. And the odd thing is, that was the extent of my injuries." He points to a bruise on his arm. "It bumped on the door when the car finally came to rest, and I got out." He looks at Eddie again, his lips together in a horizontal slice, his face and eyes still, his cane still—silent.

One. Two. Three. Four seconds.

I don't move. I don't breathe.

"Is it possible, in your attempts to stop the vehicle, you might have been pumping the accelerator?" Eddie asks.

"It's certainly something you can't overlook."

More silence. Five seconds. Russell Weller's eyes flick back and forth, from Eddie to Virginia, from Virginia to Eddie, both with their pens to the page.

"Well, do I walk out? I'll tell you, I can't drive that car. You should have seen it after I ran over a dozen apple crates and things like that."

"More like seventy-three people!" I shout. "Did you hear me? Seventy-three!"

With one dismissive phrase, "things like that," Russell Weller reduced the dozens of people he ran over to mere "things." In his sanitized version of events, his car was damaged by apple crates and other inanimate objects that got in *his* way.

Is it possible that shock erased everything he saw and heard? Similar to how my brain protected me from the devastation that followed the moment I picked up the peach, was the horror of what happened less than two hours earlier buried deep in his unconscious and inaccessible to him? Or is he simply choosing to deny what happened because he does not want to face the truth? Even worse, does he hope to mislead the police, and convince the detectives he, too, is a victim, an older driver trapped in a malfunctioning, runaway car?

One. Two seconds. A gentle tap of his cane. "God almighty." His speech slows, his voice faltering. "Those poor, poor tragic people. What a tragic ending to their outing. And I contributed to it." Sorrow seeps from the deepest, darkest center of him. I swear I hear it, the crack of a cry opening up in his throat.

I weep out loud, soaking myself in tears, and press my hand against the television screen. I want so much to reach into it, to catch the cry of wide-open grief emerging from his mouth, as if touch is the only way I can be certain this man is real and I just heard what I swear is the unmistakable sound of remorse. Then, from far down inside me, I dig desperately for a scrap of faith in his sorrow. It comes loose, and with great relief, I speak directly to him. "Thank you, thank you." I am done letting him crush me.

In that moment, I do what I must do—for myself. I forgive him.

Epilogue

Beets, cantaloupe, green beans—an abundance of color spread in a semi-circle before us like a tapestry. It is the summer of 2023, twenty years since the Santa Monica Farmers' market crash. I'm sitting next to John, playing my fiddle while he sings "Rocky Road to Dublin," a rowdy Irish song about a man who leaves his home in Galway to seek his fortune. In a way, I feel as if I have found my fortune, right here, performing at a local farmers' market. As I push my bow across the strings of the fiddle, adrenalized by the accented beats of the slip-jig, I feel safe sitting under a tent on the grass, a comfortable distance from moving cars. A preschooler with hair the color of midnight, and wearing a light-blue dress, watches us intently as she snacks on berries. A smiling woman, who could be her grandmother, stands beside the little girl, swaying side-to-side, swishing her red paisley skirt. A young teenager skips to the music, lifting her feet up high and swinging her arms. Parents holding infants join in, their sandaled feet doing a percussive dance. The farmers under their tents feel the music, too, clapping, some singing along during the chorus. Everyone here is having fun, and so am I. Four hours of uninterrupted fun.

Then comes the interruption. An older woman—in her mid-eighties, I guess—shuffles toward the roped-off gravel lot, straight toward a Buick LeSabre parked a good hundred feet to the left of where John and I were sitting just moments ago. The only apparent difference between her car and Russell Weller's car is the color. Her car is silver; his was maroon. The woman and the car are triggers: I think of how easily Russell Weller attributed the cause of the crash to his Buick. Something swells inside of me, not so much fear, but anger.

"I bet that's hers," I say to John, pointing to the car. What are the chances? Just a few weeks since the twentieth anniversary of the accident, and we're at a farmers' market, where a woman, who appears to be about the age Russell Weller was at the time of the crash, gets into the driver's seat of the Buick.

I take a deep breath, then blow the anger out in one full exhale. The anger recedes. I refuse to let it ruin the music. The music itself helps. You can't enjoy it and still have room for anger. The power of the lyrics and the melody still hums through me as we head home—a day reserved for song and dance.

I keep making music, for others and for myself, at home in my living room, the couch and rocking chair my audience. I make full bow strokes, my fingertips sliding up and down the strings, the upbeat tempo, like hyperbaric oxygen, driving out the anger and replacing it with new air. It is my fiddle that rescues me. The music is my first responder when my anger toward Russell Weller re-emerges and knocks me sideways. These days, it's usually news of yet another vehicle-ramming attack. Other times, it's news of an older driver crash: another incident of pedal confusion, of someone driving the wrong way on an interstate, or shifting into drive instead of reverse and plowing through a storefront, into a schoolyard, or along a pedestrian walkway. That's when my body remembers—the slam against the pavement, the impact crushing my pelvis, rupturing my spleen, jarring my brain. I hear the echo of Russell Weller's initial response when bystanders pulled him out of the Buick. "If you saw me coming, why didn't you get out of the way?" Then comes the lick of a flame in my gut, and I try with all my might to hold tight against the memory-punch of his deflective words: "I contributed to it," as if someone or something else were to blame. As if he hadn't been the one to run us over. That's when I ask myself, "Have I forgiven him? Will my forgiveness ever be absolute, unwavering?" I don't know. But what I do know is I still have my fiddle—and the video.

Russell Weller is gone, but I can always fast forward to the 16:53 mark, and convince myself, once again, that he was sorry.

Acknowledgements

This book—and the years spent writing it—gave me purpose and meaningful connections during a life period where I had lost my previous self and had to build a new me. It is those connections—with family, friends, mentors, and editors—that made this book possible.

My deepest thanks to environmental journalist, writing instructor, and author Alexis Lathem, who said yes to mentoring me (a novice writer) when I had no idea where to begin. It was her honest and direct feedback that pushed me to climb out of my small world in order to craft a meaningful story. I am also profoundly grateful to the Vermont College of Fine Arts (VCFA) MFA in Writing program, and to faculty members Abby Frucht, Rigoberto Gonzalez, Sascha Feinstein, and Sue William Silverman. Thank you for guiding me to convert the personal to the universal.

Loads of loving gratitude to my VCFA workshop peers and early readers, who read various iterations of chapter upon chapter with great devotion and attention. Mira Bartok, thank you for believing in this story from the beginning—and for the tough, necessary edits that helped me find its true center. Thank you to writing coach Elizabeth Cohen. *The Peach* would not be in the wide-open world without your tireless advocacy; you would not let my story remain buried in some forgotten file on my computer's hard drive. Thank you to the master of narrative journalism, Samme Chittum, whose sharp editorial eye and no-nonsense approach elevated the book in numerous ways. Your contagious enthusiasm, Samme, buoyed me when I needed it most.

Thank you to Women Writing VT for your support, Angela Palm for your insight and edits, Suzanne Nussey for your thorough proofreading, and Jacquie Kelley for your careful attention to language and inclusion.

Thank you to Sarah Cronin for your creative savvy in designing the book cover, and Laura Smyth for your smart sensitivity to the editorial design of the content.

Huge gratitude to publisher Ron Starbuck for bringing my memoir on board with Mnemosyne Books and for having faith in the importance of my story.

This book would not exist, and my life would not have continued, without those who came to my aid at the Santa Monica Farmers' Market in July 2003. My deepest gratitude to Tina Fasbender for saving my life and my destiny the moment I reached out to you from the pavement and you accepted my hand. A loving thanks to your son, now Dr. Brett Goodfriend, an emergency-room physician saving countless lives.

Thank you to the rescue workers and medical teams at Los Angeles General Medical Center, Cedars-Sinai Medical Center, and Central Vermont Medical Center for their compassion and care. Thank you to the Santa Monica Chamber of Commerce for helping me and others return to our homes and new lives. Thank you to Attorney Steven Archer for guiding me through the legal aftermath of the tragedy, and sincere gratitude to my mental health providers for your steady support.

To my dear friends—especially Kathleen, Rick, Ainsley, and Ben Burroughs—thank you for your generosity, love, and for giving me a place to land during my recovery. To my extended circle of friends and colleagues, including my NICU community at the University of Vermont Medical Center, thank you for your care and encouragement.

To Eric, and all my family, thank you for your constant presence, advocacy, and love as I found my way forward toward healing. Mom, I love you a lot. A mother's love surpasses all others in our healing journeys.

And finally, to my best friend and husband, John. From reading early excerpts to editing, proofreading, and listening to me hem and haw about what I should and should not delete, you were as important to the completion of *The Peach* as I was. John, thank you for being my true polestar.

Source Notes

PRELUDE

The number of people who died (...the day ten people died...) was verified from the relevant National Transportation Safety Board *Highway Accident Report* and also newspaper reports: Rubin, Joel, et al. "Car Plows through Crowd in Santa Monica, Killing 9." *Los Angeles Times*, 17 July 2003, p. A1. Molloy, Tim. "Infant Is 10th Fatality in Market Accident." *The Burlington Free Press*, 18 July 2003, p. 5A. National Transportation Safety Board (NTSB). *Highway Accident Report: Rear End Collision and Subsequent Vehicle Intrusion into Pedestrian Space at Certified Farmers' Market Santa Monica, California July 16, 2003.* NTSB/HAR-04/04. Washington, DC. 3 Aug. 2004, "Executive Summary," p.vi.

CHAPTER 1

Descriptive details about the accident (I do not remember...) are sourced in Prologue, "Car Plows through Crowd in Santa Monica, Killing 9."

Specific details regarding the accident (...bumper catching a little girl...) were drawn from Mohan, Geoffrey. "Suddenly, They Were Gone." *Los Angeles Times,* 19 July 2003, p. A28.

The quote, "My baby. My baby," was verified from news report: Hoffman, Allison, et al. "A Whirlwind for Rescuers and Hospitals." *Los Angeles Times*, 19 July 2003, p. B1.

Descriptive details of the accident scene (...Buick racing...people splayed...a woman trapped...) are sourced in Prologue, "Car Plows through Crowd in Santa Monica, Killing 9."

CHAPTER 2

Details regarding the age of victims, their injuries and names (. . . seven-month-old Brandon David Esfahani was bleeding . . .) were verified using newspaper reports and court documents: See Chapter 1, "A Whirlwind for Rescuers and Hospitals." Sionit, Mojdeh. "Persian Jews Mourn Deaths at Market." *Jewish Journal*, 24 July 2003, www.jewishjournal.com/community/8172/. Accessed 8 Mar. 2024. Also, The Farmers' Market Plaintiffs' Steering Committee. "Release of All Claims," Exhibit "B."

Age and injuries of victims (...fifty-year-old Kevin McCarthy, bleeding...) were verified using various newspaper reports: See Chapter 1, "A Whirlwind for Rescuers and Hospitals."

Age and injuries of victims (...eighty-nine-year-old Shamsi Khani, the oldest survivor...) were verified from various newspaper reports, including: Groves, Martha. "Market Survivor 'a Miracle.'" *Los Angeles Times*, 27 Sep. 2003, p. B1.

Age and injuries (…twenty-five-year-old Jenna Edwards…) were verified from various newspaper reports: See Prologue, "Car Plows through Crowd in Santa Monica, Killing 9." Groves, Martha, and Anna Gorman. "Victims, Survivors, Relive Horrors." *Los Angeles Times*, 5 Dec. 2003. B9.

Spelling of the name Sandra Bacall was verified via the Sandra Bacall website: www.sandrabacall.com/. Accessed 5 Feb. 2026. Her age (forty-seven) and injuries were verified from the following newspaper report: "Eleven New Suits Filed in Market Tragedy." *Santa Monica Daily Free Press,* 14 June 2004, vol. 3, no. 209, p. 6.

Injuries and ages of victims (…sixty-year-old Ilona Lettrich…) were verified from news reports: See "Victims, Survivors, Relive Horrors." Verification of injuries: Spano, John, and Groves, Martha. "Felony Manslaughter Verdict for Driver in Market Crash." *Los Angeles Times*, 21 Oct. 2006, p. A16. First news story reports two fingers nearly severed.

Injuries of victim Bartley Bard were verified from news report: Hunt, Stephen. "Bards Back for Lunch." *Calgary Herald*, 11 Nov. 2006. "California Crash Injured Calgary Theatre Co-Founder." *The Globe and Mail,* 18 Apr. 2018. Also see "Victims, Survivors, Relive Horrors." Verification of Bard's age, (…sixty-one…) Radaris People Finder 360. www.radaris.com/ng/search?ff=Bartley&fl=Bard&fs=Canada. Accessed 8 Mar. 2024.

The age of the driver of the car that struck pedestrians at the Farmers' Market (…eighty-six-year-old…) is sourced in Prologue, NTSB. "Executive Summary," p. vi.

CHAPTER 4

Names and ages of victims were verified from Plaintiffs' Steering Committee "Release of All Claims" and also newspaper reports: Winton, Richard and Martha Groves. "Case Is Closed on Deadly Day at Market." *Los Angeles Times*, 22 May 2008, www.latimes.com/archives/la-xpm-2008-may-22-me-market22-story.html. Accessed 26 Feb. 2025. "Mount Sinai Memorial Park in Hollywood Hills, California, Find a Grave Cemetery," www.findagrave.com/memorial/16722626/molok-ghoulian-nabatian Accessed 3 April. 2026. Winton, Richard and Martha Groves. "Santa Monica Settles Crash Lawsuits." *Los Angeles Times,* 22 May 2008, p. A21. Spano, John. "Ruling Lets Victims of Farmers Market Crash Sue Santa Monica." *Los Angeles Times*, 17 Oct. 2007, p. B3. Rubin, Joel. "With Few Clues Market Crash Victim Remained a Mystery." *Los Angeles Times*, 23 July 2003, p. B1. Spano, John. "Driver In Crash That Killed 10 'Looked Angry.'" *Los Angeles Times,* 15 Sept. 2006, p. B4. Also see "Exhibit 'A' and 'B'", Release of All Claims.

CHAPTER 10

Details about the preventable causes of related accidents (…pedal error…) were verified from multiple sources: See Prologue, NTSB *Highway Accident Report*, pp. 35-39. Also: Admin. "Pedal Error Causing Preventable Accidents." *Claims Journal*, Wells Media Group Network, 17 July 2015, www.claimsjournal.com/news/national/2015/07/17/264606.htm. Accessed 15 Feb. 2026.

Details about a 1992 accident (...1992 field trip turned horror...) were verified from McRoberts, Flynn, et al. "Field-Trip Horror: Car Plows into Kids." *Chicago Tribune*, 10 Aug. 2021, www.chicagotribune.com/1992/05/01/field-trip-horror-car-plows-into-kids/. Accessed 15 Feb. 2026.

Relevant details and the date (...August 2012...) of an accident involving an older driver and pedestrians were verified from news report: Vives, Ruben and Robert J Lopez. "Driver, 100, Hits 11 Near School." *Los Angeles Times*, 30 Aug. 2012, pp. AA1 – AA5.

Details about a multiple casualty 2019 accident in Kyodo, Japan involving an elderly driver (...in April 2019...) were verified from news report: "Two Feared Dead, Eight Injured After Elderly Driver Plows Car into Pedestrians in Tokyo." *The Straits Times*, 20 April 2019, www.straitstimes.com/asia/east-asia/10-people-injured-2-critically-after-car-plows-into-pedestrians-in-tokyo. Accessed 16 Feb. 2026.

Details about a 2025 accident involving an older driver (...in April 2025...) were verified from the following article: Staff Reports. "Elderly Woman Dies Following Three-Vehicle Crash in Pike County, Ohio." *Eyewitness News, WCHS Fox*, 21 Apr. 2025, wchstv.com/news/local/elderly-woman-killed-following-three-vehicle-crash-in-pike-county-ohio. Accessed 27 Dec. 2025.

CHAPTER 12

Details about a 2016 vehicle-ramming attack in Nice, France (A man had rented a cargo truck...) was verified from news report: "Nice Attack: What We Know About the Bastille Day Killings." *BBC News*, BBC, 19 Aug. 2016, www.bbc.com/news/world-europe-36801671. Accessed 17 Feb. 2026.

List of vehicle-ramming attacks (If you type in "vehicle-ramming...) were verified from the following online encyclopedia: "Vehicle-Ramming Attack," *Wikipedia*, Wikimedia Foundation, 6 Nov. 2025, en.wikipedia.org/wiki/Vehicle-ramming_attack#Causes_and_motives. Accessed 17 Feb. 2026.

Details about a 2018 vehicle-ramming incident in Toronto, Canada (The city is safe...) were verified from news report: Rumley, Jonathan. "10 Dead, 14 Injured After Van Hits Pedestrians in Toronto." *Yahoo News*, Yahoo, 23 Apr. 2018, ca.news.yahoo.com/toronto-fire-says-numerous-casualties-vehicle-hits-crowd-182502742.html. Accessed 18 Feb. 2026.

Details about a driver of a 2018 Toronto vehicle-ramming incident (Minassian – a twenty-year-old college student...) were verified from news report: Laidlaw, Katherine. "The Man Behind the Yonge Street Van Attack." *Toronto Life*, 22 Apr. 2019, torontolife.com/city/man-behind-yonge-street-van-attack/. Accessed 18 Feb. 2026.

Details about the Santa Monica Farmers' Market memorial event (...service for all those who died...) were verified from news report: Williams, Erica. "Santa Monica Mourns One Week After Market Tragedy." *Santa Monica Lookout News*, 23 July 2003, www.surfsantamonica.com/ssm_site/the_lookout/news/News-2003/July-2003/07_24_03_Santa_Monica_Mourns.htm. Accessed 18 Feb. 2026.

Details about memorial services held for victims of the Farmers' Market crash (Other, small services were held.) were verified from Facebook: Lynne Weaver Memorial. "About Lynne Weaver Memorial." *Facebook*, 16 July 2011, www.facebook.com/p/Lynne-Weaver-Memorial-100064614432181/. Accessed 26 Mar. 2026.

Details about memorial services held for victims of the Farmers' Market crash (On July 21, Diana and Kevin were remembered...) is sourced in Chapter 1, "Suddenly, They Were Gone."

Details about the film (*The Rogue Shoes*) were verified from Internet Database: Gong, David, et al. *The Rogue Shoes.* Performance by Marisa Petroro, et al., Plate-O-Shrimp Productions, 2004, www.imdb.com/title/tt0423092/?ref_=wl_li_tt. Accessed 30 Mar. 2026.

Details about memorial service held for Brandon and Molok (Some 750 attended their funeral.) are sourced in Chapter 2, "Persian Jews Mourn Deaths."

Details about deceased victim Theresa Breglia (...investigators released the name...) are sourced in Chapter 4, "With Few Clues."

CHAPTER 13

Details about barriers in place at the time of the Farmers' Market crash (...only plastic orange-and-white striped barriers...) are sourced in Prologue, NTSB. *Highway Accident Report*, p. 40.

Russell Weller's current and past health history (Blood samples taken...) is sourced in Prologue, NTSB. *Highway Accident Report*, p. 7.

Russell Weller's driving history (Though he had no moving violations...) is sourced in Prologue, NTSB. *Highway Accident Report*, p. 5.

Russell Weller's activities before speeding through the Farmers' Market (...Weller stopped to mail a letter...) are sourced in Prologue, NTSB. *Highway Accident Report*, p. 7.

CHAPTER 15

The quote, "I accidentally killed her," was taken from the following book: Kidd, Sue Monk. "Chapter Twelve." *Secret Life of Bees.* New York, Penguin, 2003. P. 242.

Descriptive details about the accident (Maybe Cindy's mother wished...) are sourced in Chapter 1, "Suddenly, They Were Gone."

Descriptive details about the accident (Maybe Brandon's mother regretted...) are sourced in Chapter 4, "Case is Closed on Deadly Day at Market."

Descriptive details about the accident (And maybe Lynne's husband...) are sourced in Chapter 1, "Suddenly, They Were Gone."

Specifics about victims of Nice, France vehicle-ramming attack (Russell Schulz later joined my yellow world.) were verified from news report: "'He Didn't Destroy Me. We Carry On. He Lost': Survivors of Terror Attacks Look Back." *The Guardian*, Guardian News and Media, 25 May 2019, www.theguardian.com/cities/2019/may/25/life-after-death-survivors-of-terror-attacks. Accessed 18 Feb. 2026.

CHAPTER 16

Middle name of Lily (... Lily's middle name was Melissa.) is sourced in Chapter 15, *Secret Life of Bees*, p. 41.

CHAPTER 19

The quote, "thrashing," and the descriptive details of Jenna's flashbacks (Jenna, a budding actress...) were verified from the following online magazine: "Meet Jenna Edwards of Create Your Life." *Voyage LA*, 13 Nov. 2017, www.voyagela.com/interview/meet-jenna-edwards-createyourlife-ive-burbank-16-years-start-year-long-voyage-traveling-across-us-teardrop-trailer-husband-dog/. Accessed 18 Feb. 2026.

Descriptive details of Shamsi's flashbacks (Shamsi's dreams...) were verified from news report: Groves, Martha. "Market Survivor 'Is a 'Miracle.'" *Los Angeles Times*, 27 Sept. 2003, p. B16.

The quote, "the carnage of humanity...," and the descriptive details of Sandra's flashbacks (Sandra's dreams...) were verified via the Sandra Bacall website page: www.sandrabacall.com/bio.html. Accessed 18 Mar. 2026.

Date and details (In December 2016...) of Berlin, Germany vehicle-ramming attack were verified from news reports: Huggler, Justin. "German Police Warned Anis Amri Was Planning a Suicide Attack Nine Months Before Berlin Christmas Market Massacre." *Telegraph.Co*, The Telegraph, 26 Mar. 2017, www.telegraph.co.uk/news/2017/03/26/german-police-warned-anis-amri-planning-suicide-attack-nine/. Accessed 18 Feb. 2026.

Date and details (In December 2024...) of German market attack were verified from news report: Simon, Scott and Rebecca Collard. "Car Plows into Crowd at German Christmas Market." *Weekend Edition*, National Public Radio, WUSF, Tampa, 21 Dec. 2024, www.npr.org/2024/12/21/nx-s1-5235526/car-plows-into-crowds-at-german-christmas-market. Accessed 18 Feb. 2026.

The quote, "Boom, boom," was verified from news report: Winter, Tom, et al. "Car Rams into Pedestrians in NYC's Times Square, Killing at Least 1." *NBC News*, 19 May 2017, www.nbcnews.com/news/us-news/car-rams-pedestrians-nyc-s-times-square-n761556. Accessed 26 Mar. 2026.

The quote, "massive bang," was verified from news report: Connolly, Kate. "Berlin Attack: Officials Fear That Armed Perpetrator is Still on the Loose." *The Guardian*, 20 Dec. 2016, www.theguardian.com/world/2016/dec/20/police-uncertain-they-have-suspect-in-berlin-christmas-market-attack. Accessed 26 Mar. 2026.

The quote, "reminiscent of a war," was verified from news report: Guardian staff and agencies. "Deadly Christmas Market Car Attack in Germany: What We Know So Far." *The Guardian,* 20 Dec. 2024, www.theguardian.com/world/2024/dec/21/deadly-christmas-market-car-attack-in-germany-what-we-know-so-far. Accessed 26 Mar. 2026.

CHAPTER 20

Description of Russell Weller's emotional state (Russell Weller's identity tattoo . . .) after the Farmers' Market crash was verified from news report: Gorman, Anna. "Market Tragedy Took Driver's Spirit, Kin Say." *Los Angeles Times,* 5 Jan. 2004, www.latimes.com/archives/la-xpm-2004-jan-05-me-weller5-story.html. Accessed 26 Mar. 2026.

CHAPTER 23

The quote, "Car Plows through Crowd," is sourced in Prologue, "Car Plows through Crowd in Santa Monica, Killing 9."

CHAPTER 26

The quote, "George Russell Weller has not been charged with a crime," can be found in the following radio broadcast: Grotsky, Joe. Interview with Nova Safo. "'Older Motorists Head Back to Drivers' Safety Classes,'" *All Things Considered*, National Public Radio, KPCC, Los Angeles, 24 Sept. 2003, www.npr.org/2003/09/24/1444902/older-motorists-head-back-to-drivers-ed-class. Accessed 16 Feb. 2026.

The quotes, "I've been driving for seventy-five years... my reaction time isn't that bad... lucky," are sourced in "Older Motorists Head Back to Drivers' Safety Classes."

The paraphrased quote, (When Grotsky says...) is sourced in "Older Motorists Head Back to Drivers' Safety Classes."

Details of Vermont's public transit (Entombed in our country's poor public transportation system...) can be found in the following op-ed: Poor, Kelly S. "Don't Leave Older Vermonters Stranded," 17 Feb. 2026, vtdigger.org/2026/02/17/kelly-stoddard-poor-dont-leave-older-vermonters-stranded/. Accessed 26 Mar. 2026.

Details of claim regarding Russell Weller's health (... his uncle had suffered...) are sourced in Chapter 20, "Market Tragedy Took Driver's Spirit, Kin Say."

Details of Russell Weller's health (He was awake and alert...) is sourced in Prologue, NTSB, *Highway Accident Report*, p. 33.

The quote, "Grotsky plans to turn off...," is sourced in "Older Motorists Head Back to Drivers' Safety Classes."

CHAPTER 27

The quote, "The Lord said to Eli'phaz...," can be found in Bible excerpt: Job: 42:17. *The Holy Bible: Revised Standard Version with Apocrypha*. 50th ed., Oxford University Press, 2002.

CHAPTER 28

Details of car (Was it a lesson God couldn't wait to teach when a Dodge Challenger...) used in 2017 Charlottesville attack were verified from the online encyclopedia page: *Wikipedia*, Wikimedia Foundation, 12 Feb. 2026, en.wikipedia.org/wiki/Charlottesville_car_attack. Accessed 19 Feb 2026.

Details of 2017 Charlottesville attack (An avowed white supremacist...) were verified from news report: Wamsley, Laurel and Allyn, Bobby. "Neo-Nazi Who Killed Charlottesville Protester Is Sentenced to Life in Prison," *NPR*, 28 Aug. 2019, www.npr.org/2019/06/28/736915323/neo-nazi-who-killed-charlottesville-protester-is-sentenced-to-life-in-prison. Accessed 19 Feb 2026.

The following quotes, "Jews will not replace us... Blood and soil," and the details of the 2017 Charlottesville attack were verified from the following op-ed: Ruttenberg, Danya. "Why Do White Supremacists Hate Jews? Because We Can Fight Them," *Chicago Tribune,* 11 Aug. 2019, www.chicagotribune.com/2017/08/17/why-do-white-supremacists-hate-jews-because-we-can-fight-them/. Accessed 19 Feb. 2026. Also: Fieldstadt, Elisha. "James Alex Fields, Driver in Deadly Car Attack at Charlottesville Rally, Sentenced to Life in Prison," *NBCNews.com*, NBCUniversal News Group, 28 June 2019, www.nbcnews.com/news/us-news/james-alex-fields-driver-deadly-car-attack-charlottesville-rally-sentenced-n1024436. Accessed 19 Feb. 2026.

The quote, "White lives matter," was verified from news report: "Charlottesville Attack: What, Where and Who?" *Al Jazeera*, Al Jazeera Media Network, 17 Aug 2017, www.aljazeera.com/news/2017/8/17/charlottesville-attack-what-where-and-who. Accessed 19 Feb. 2026.

Number of people killed (Ten also died in the 2018 Toronto vehicle-ramming attack.) in Toronto attack was verified from news report: CBS News. "Portraits of the Toronto Van Attack," *CBC Radio Canada,* 2018, newsinteractives.cbc.ca/longform-custom/lives-remembered/. Accessed 19 Mar. 2026.

CHAPTER 30

Details about the preventable causes of related accidents are sourced in Prologue, NTSB. *Highway Accident Report.* Also see Chapter 10, "Pedal Error Causing Preventable Accidents."

Details of who is at risk (...it's far more likely to happen to people in two age groups...) of pedal error are sourced in Chapter 10, "Pedal Error Causing Preventable Accidents."

Details of a 2021 Tulsa, Oklahoma crash (It happened in Tulsa...) were verified from news report: "Car Crashes into Arby's Restaurant in Tulsa," *2 News Oklahoma KJRH Tulsa,* 13 Apr. 2021, www.kjrh.com/news/local-news/car-crashes-into-arbys-restaurant-in tulsa#:~:text=The%20driver%20crashed%20into%20the,drive%2Dthru%20will%20remain%20open. Accessed 19 May 2026.

Details of a 2018 Dallas crash (It happened in Dallas...) were verified from news report: Sang, Lucia S. "Car Plows into Dallas-Area Metro PCS Store, Hits Woman," *Fox News*, 27 Mar. 2018, www.foxnews.com/us/car-plows-into-dallas-area-metro-pcs-store-hits-woman. Accessed 5 May 2024.

CHAPTER 34

Definition of "repetition compulsion" was verified from the following book: Celani, David P. "Introduction." *Leaving Home*. Colombia University Press, Columbia, New York, NY, 2005. P. 10.

CHAPTER 38

Details of Eye Movement Desensitization Reprocessing (The PTSD therapist I started seeing . . .) were verified from the EMDR Institute website: "EMDR." What is EMDR. EMDR Therapy is an Eight-phase Treatment," EMDR Institute, Inc., 2026, www.emdr.com/what-is-emdr/. Accessed 19 Feb. 2026.

Details about complex PTSD (...she explains that I likely have...) were verified from the Cleveland Clinic website: "Complex PTSD," *Cleveland Clinic*, 2 Oct. 2025, my.clevelandclinic.org/health/diseases/24881-cptsd-complex-ptsd. Accessed 19 Feb. 2026.

Details about memory conformity (I experienced a kind of...) were verified from the following online encyclopedia page: "Memory Conformity." *Wikipedia*, Wikimedia Foundation, 28 Sept. 2025, en.wikipedia.org/wiki/Memory_conformity#cite_note-Valentine-3. Accessed 19 Feb. 2026. Also: Roediger, Henry L., et al. "Social Contagion of Memory," *Psychonomic Bulletin & Review*, A Journal of the Psychonomic Society, Springer Nature, vol. 8, no. 2, 2001, pp. 365 – 371.

CHAPTER 42

Details about pedal-error incidents (Each time I learn of any driver...) were verified from news reports: WWL Staff. "Car Plunges off Rooftop Parking Garage, Crashes into Shopping Center," *WWLTV.com*, 27 Feb. 2017, www.khou.com/article/news/car-plunges-off-rooftop-parking-garage-crashes-into-shopping-center-below/285-414843287. Accessed 27 Mar. 2026. Also see: Geanous, Jacob. "Woman Mistakes Brakes for Gas and Drives into River," *Metro*, Associated Newspapers Limited, 17 July 2019, metro.co.uk/2019/07/17/woman-mistakes-brakes-gas-drives-car-river-10392567/. Accessed 19 July 2026.

CHAPTER 43

Descriptive details of Jenna's recovery (Jenna, a budding actress...) are sourced in Chapter 19, "Meet Jenna Edwards of Create Your Life."

Details regarding Jenna's acting and personal background (...*Buffy the Vampire Slayer*...abuse...poverty...eating disorder...no longer suffer...) were verified from the following webpage: "Jenna Edwards Biography," www.imdb.com/name/nm1173971/. Accessed 27 Mar. 2026. Also, Jenna Edwards website, www.jennaedwards.com/about-jenna. Accessed 27 Mar. 2026. Jenna's background is also sourced in Chapter 19, "Meet Jenna Edwards of Create Your Life."

Details regarding Bartley's recovery (...traumatic brain injury...screenwriter...*The Golden Hour*...) were verified from news article: Louis Hobson. "Play Personal for Calgary Theatre Man and His Struggle to Get His Life Back," *Calgary Sun*, 21 June 2011.

Details regarding Shamsi's recovery (...one leg shorter...unable to stand...) were verified from news article: Groves, Martha. "A New Sense of Loss at Farmers Market," *Los Angeles Times*, 16 Sept. 2006, www.latimes.com/archives/la-xpm-2006-sep-16-me-market16-story.html. Accessed 27 Mar. 2026.

Details regarding Sandra's recovery (Sandra...injured foot...*Ghost Town Café*.) were verified from Spotify: Bacall, Sandra. *Ghost Town Café*, 2006, www.sandrabacall.com/bio.html. Spotify, open.spotify.com/album/02mc86nWj6fNUcYPlp6y49. Accessed 27 Mar. 2026. Also: Bacall, Sandra. *Ghost Town Cafe*. *Pandora*, Pandora Media, LLC, 2006, www.pandora.com/artist/sandra-bacall/ghost-town-cafe/ALdp9jnzjxtgknZ. Accessed 19 Feb. 2026. Injuries sourced in Chapter 2, "Eleven New Suits Filed in Market Tragedy."

Details regarding Russell Weller's manslaughter charges (...ten counts...pleaded not guilty...) were verified from news reports: Gorman, Anna. "Driver Who Killed 10 Is Charged," *Los Angeles Times*, 6 Jan. 2004, pp. B1–B8. Also: Lookout Staff. "Weller Pleads Not Guilty in Santa Monica Crash," *Santa Monica LookOut News*, 8 Dec. 2004, www.surfsantamonica.com/ssm_site/the_lookout/news/News-2004/Dec-2004/12_08_04_Weller_Pleads_Not_Guilty.htm. Accessed 27 Mar. 2026.

For details regarding Russell Weller's plea in court (At a December 2004 hearing . . .) see "Weller Pleads Not Guilty in Santa Monica Crash."

The quotes, "pedal error," "error in response execution," and "comparatively common," are sourced in Prologue, NTSB. *Highway Accident Report*, "Analysis," pp. 36–38.

The quote, "Hitting the accelerator instead of the brake...," was taken from news report: "Manslaughter Charges Stand Against Driver, 88," *The Spokesman Review*, 20 Mar. 2005, www.spokesman.com/stories/2005/mar/20/goodfellas-figure-faces-drug-charge/. Accessed 23 Feb. 2026.

CHAPTER 44

Details regarding executive-function testing (The average thirty-something-year-old can name forty-three words.) were verified from the following journal: Tombaugh, T, et al. "Normative Data Stratified by Age and Education for Two Measures of Verbal Fluency Fas and Animal Naming," *Archives of Clinical Neuropsychology*, vol. 14, no. 2, Feb. 1999, pp. 167–177.

Details regarding neuroplasticity (But after reading the latest research...) were verified from the Brain Line website: Campbell, Celeste. "What Is Neuroplasticity?" *BrainLine*, 26 July 2018, www.brainline.org/author/celeste-campbell/qa/what-neuroplasticity. Accessed 23 Feb. 2026.

CHAPTER 45

Details regarding Memory and Attention Adaptation Training (She calls the exercises... MAAT...) can be found in the following research article: Ferguson, Robert J, and Amber A Martinson. "An Overview of Cognitive-Behavioral Management of Memory Dysfunction Associated with Chemotherapy," *Psicooncologia*, 2011. vol. 8, no. 2-3, pp. 385-404.

Unable to obtain permission to share details of MAAT manual. Recent research regarding data about traumatic brain injuries can be found via the Center for Brain Injury and Repair. "Traumatic Brain Injury: A 'Silent Epidemic,'" *Perelman School of Medicine at the University of Pennsylvania*, www.med.upenn.edu/cbir/silentepidemic.html. Accessed 27 Mar. 2026.

Details regarding the phrase, "invisible disability," were verified through various online resources, including the following: "Brain Injury as a Form of Invisible Disability," *Brain Injury Association of America*, 25 June 2024, biausa.org/public-affairs/media/brain-injury-as-a-form-of-invisible-disability. Accessed 27 Mar. 2026.

Details regarding Bartley's recovery (While at a party...) are sourced in Chapter 43, "Play Personal for Calgary Theatre Man and His Struggle to Get His Life Back."

CHAPTER 46

Details regarding meaning of *Timshel* can be found in the following novel: Steinbeck, John. "24." *East of Eden*, Penguin Books, London, 2002, p. 303

The quote, "thou mayest," is sourced in *East of Eden*.

CHAPTER 47

Reference to where Shamsi was standing (... near Second Street...) at the time of the Farmers' Market crash is sourced in Chapter 43, "A New Sense of Loss at Farmers Market."

Descriptive details of Shamsi (... newspaper photo of a woman... Shamsi was a caretaker.) are sourced in Chapter 2, "Market Survivor 'A Miracle.'"

Details regarding the death of Shamsi, and the quote, "Shamsi Khani, ninety-two, the oldest victim of the 2003 crash dies..." are both sourced in Chapter 43, "A New Sense of Loss at Farmers Market."

The epitaph, "Shamsi Maman Khani... Beloved matriarch, mother, grandmother, and great-grandmother," was verified from the following website: "Mount Sinai Memorial Park in Hollywood Hills, California, Find a Grave Cemetery," *Find a Grave*, www.findagrave.com/memorial/109719991/shamsi-khani. Accessed 27 Mar. 2026.

Details of Shamsi's last visit to the Farmers' Market (... she chose Asian pears...) are sourced in Chapter 43, "A New Sense of Loss at Farmers Market."

The quotes, "I have also written about that day... How do we speak...", were taken from an email exchange: Bacall, Sandra. Received by Melissa Cronin, 24 Aug. 2009.

The quote, "Her famous shoe...," is sourced in email exchange: Bacall, Sandra. Received by Melissa Cronin. Also see Chapter 19, Sandra Bacall website page: www.sandrabacall.com/bio.html. Accessed 27 Mar. 2026.

CHAPTER 48

The quotes, "I couldn't believe what I was seeing... He was hitting people...," are sourced in Prologue, "Car Plows through Crowd in Santa Monica, Killing 9."

The quote, "Boom! Boom! Boom!" is sourced in Prologue, "Car Plows through Crowd in Santa Monica, Killing 9."

The quote, "How many people did I hit?" is sourced in Prologue, "Car Plows through Crowd in Santa Monica, Killing 9," p. A14.

The quote, "If you saw me coming...," is sourced in Lookout Staff. "Weller Found Guilty in Market Crash," Santa Monica Lookout News, 20 Oct. 2006, www.surfsantamonica.com/ssm_site/the_lookout/news/News-2006/October-2006/10_20_06_Weller_Found_Guilty_in_Market_Crash.htm. Accessed 27 Mar. 2026.

Reference to Russell Weller mailing a letter (... let the postman...) was verified from the following recorded interview: Weller, George R. Interview. Conducted by Eddie Chavez. 16 July 2003. "Santa Monica Police Department Interview of George Russell Weller." DVD 2003.

The quotes, "I know it wasn't an accident... he did it on purpose... he hit everything he could," are sourced in Chapter 2, "Victims, Survivors, Relive Horrors."

The quote, "murderer," is sourced in Prologue, "Car Plows through Crowd in Santa Monica, Killing 9."

The quote, "coward," was verified from news report: Spano, John, and Martha Groves. "No Prison for Weller, No Closure for Others." *Los Angeles Times*, 21 Nov. 2006, www.latimes.com/archives/la-xpm-2006-nov-21-me-weller21-story.html. Accessed. 26 Feb. 2026.

CHAPTER 49

Details regarding (How much easier it would have been...) Prince Philip's 2017 car accident were verified from news report: Pérez-Peña, Richard. "Prince Philip, 97, Won't Face Charges Over Car Crash, Prosecutors Say." *The New York Times*, 15 Feb. 2019, p. A5.

Details regarding Japan's growing population (...one of the fastest aging nations on Earth...) of older drivers were verified from news article: Lufkin, Bryan. "How Japan Is Handling More Ageing Drivers," *BBC*, 27 Oct. 2019, www.bbc.com/worklife/article/20191025-how-japan-is-handling-more-ageing-drivers. Accessed 25 Feb. 2026.

The increase in the number of older drivers in Japan (...nearly 8 million in 2003 to roughly 20 million in 2023...) was verified from the following report: World Economic Forum. "What an Ageing World Can Learn from Japan's Campaign to Get Seniors Driving Safely," *World Economic Forum*, 12 Dec. 2024, www.weforum.org/stories/2024/12/japan-senior-driver-safety/. Accessed 25 Feb. 2026.

Government response to Japan's (Those who are seventy-five and older...) increase in number of older drivers was verified from news article: "Driver's License Renewal Center for Elderly Opens in Saitama," *The Japan Times*, 12 June 2024, japannews.yomiuri.co.jp/society/general-news/20240612-191439/ Accessed 28 Mar. 2026. Also: Parry, Richard L. "Japan's Deadly Struggle: The Campaign to Get Dangerous Elderly Motorists off the Road," *The Times*, 23 June 2024. www.thetimes.com/world/asia/article/japans-deadly-struggle-the-campaign-to-get-dangerous-elderly-motorists-off-the-road-zk2fnvrc8#:~:text=Businesses%20have%20offered%20incentives%20to,of%20undertakers%20offering%20cheap%20funerals. Accessed 25 Feb. 2026.

Details regarding outcome of a 2012 pedal-error incident in Japan (...a widower from the United Kingdom...) were verified from news report: Brooks-Dutton, Ben. "My Wife Was Killed by an Older Driver. That's Why I'm Fighting for Tests," *The Guardian*, 18 Apr. 2017, www.theguardian.com/commentisfree/2017/apr/18/wife-killed-older-driver-law-change. Accessed 29 Mar. 2026

Details regarding license renewal requirements in the U.K. (...The Secretary of State...) were verified from the following: Service, Government Digital. "Renew Your Driving Licence If You're 70 or Over," *GOV.UK*, 4 Dec. 2014, www.gov.uk/renew-driving-licence-at-70. Accessed 25 Feb. 2026.

The quotes, "Voluntarily surrendering your driving license...medical condition or something else...," are sourced in "Renew Your Driving Licence If You're 70 or Over."

Details regarding 1992 older-driver (...Stella Maychick...) car crash in Washington Square Park were verified from the following blog: Komanoff, Charles. "Twenty Years Later, Horrific Washington Square Park Crash Still Resonates." *Streetsblog NYC*, 23 Apr. 2012, nyc.streetsblog.org/2012/04/23/twenty-years-later-horrific-washington-square-park-crash-still-resonates/. Accessed 25 Feb. 2026. Also see: Frank, Ted. "1995 Washington Square Sudden Acceleration Revisited." *Overlawyered*, Cato Institute, 17 Mar. 2010, www.overlawyered.com/2010/03/1995-washington-square-sudden-acceleration-revisited/. Accessed 28 Mar. 2026.

CHAPTER 50

The quoted passage, "A judge attacked George Russell Weller... 'I will place him on probation...'" is sourced in Chapter 48, "No Prison for Weller, No Closure for Others."

The quotes, "Weller has never once expressed... stubborn... bullheaded..." are sourced in Chapter 48, "No Prison for Weller, No Closure for Others."

Details regarding conviction of Russell Weller (... guilty on ten felony...) were verified from news report: Spano, John, and Martha Groves. "Driver Guilty of Felony in Market Crash," 21 Oct. 2006, www.latimes.com/archives/la-xpm-2006-oct-21-me-weller21-story.html#:~:text=In%20January%202004%2C%20Los%20Angeles,vehicular%20manslaughter%20with%20gross%20negligence. Accessed 28 Mar. 2006.

Definition of "Felony" was taken from the following online encyclopedia page: *Wikipedia*, Wikimedia Foundation, 18 Feb. 2026, en.wikipedia.org/wiki/Felony. Accessed 26 Feb. 2026.

Definition of "Gross negligence" was taken from the following online encyclopedia page: *Wikipedia*, Wikimedia Foundation, 6 July 2024, en.wikipedia.org/wiki/Gross negligence. Accessed 26 Feb. 2026.

Details regarding Russell Weller's conviction (... eighteen years in prison... more than $100,000...) were verified from news report: Barco, Mandalit del. "Jury Convicts Elderly California Driver of Manslaughter." *NPR*, 21 Nov. 2006, www.npr.org/2006/11/21/6517857/jury-convicts-elderly-california-driver-of-manslaughter. Accessed 26 Feb. 2026.

Details of reactions from families (Lynne's daughter... Shamsi's granddaughter... Movsha's daughter...) of deceased victims regarding Russell Weller's conviction are sourced in Chapter 48, "No Prison for Weller, No Closure for Others."

Details of the Farmers' Market crash settlement (... $21 million... worst pedestrian accidents...) are sourced in Chapter 4: "Case Is Closed on Deadly Day at Market."

Details regarding improved safety measures (Three years after the settlement... dragnets...) after the Farmers' Market crash were verified from news report: Groves, Martha. "Santa Monica to Use Vehicle Safety Nets at Farmers' Market." *Los Angeles Times*, 5 May 2011, www.latimes.com/local/la-xpm-2011-may-05-la-me-farmers-market-dragnets-20110503-story.html. Accessed 29 Mar. 2026.

Details regarding a 2013 pedestrian accident (There would be more to come...) were verified from news report: Chappell, Bill. "Monster Truck Crash Kills Eight at Outdoor Event in Mexico." *NPR*, 6 Oct. 2013, www.npr.org/sections/thetwo-way/2013/10/06/229872550/monster-truck-crash-kills-eight-at-outdoor-event-in-mexico. Accessed 26 Feb. 2026.

Details regarding an Austin, Texas pedestrian accident (Less than six months later...) were verified from news report: Hogan, Marc. "Revisiting the Car Crash That Shook SXSW, Two Years Later." *Pitchfork*, 16 Mar. 2016, pitchfork.com/thepitch/1057-revisiting-the-car-crash-that-shook-sxsw-two-years-later/. Accessed 26 Feb. 2026.

Details regarding a 2025 pedestrian accident (...thirty-seven-year-old woman...) were verified from news report: Liddell, James. "Minivan Plows into Festival Crowd Leaving Boy Fighting for Life and Injuring Two More." *The Independent*, 2 Sept. 2025, www.the-independent.com/news/world/americas/crime/kipona-festival-crash-driver-arrest-b2818285.html. Accessed 26 Feb. 2026.

Details regarding vehicle-ramming attacks (The escalation...from 2014 onward...) were verified from news report: Jenkins, Brian Michael, and Bruce R Butterworth. "An Analysis of Vehicle Ramming Attacks." *Transweb.Sjsu.Edu*, San Jose State University, Nov. 2019, transweb.sjsu.edu/sites/default/files/SP-1119-RB-Vehicle-Ramming-Attacks.pdf. Accessed 26 Feb. 2026.

Details regarding a 2018 pedestrian safety project (...approved $1.3 million to erect removable steel bollards...) in San Luis Obispo were verified from news report: Johnson Peter. "SLO City Council Signs Off on Downtown Bollards Project." *News Times San Luis Obispo*, 22 Feb. 2018, www.newtimesslo.com/slo-city-council-signs-off-on-downtown-bollards-project-4329538/. Accessed 28 Feb. 2026.

Details regarding a New York City vehicle-ramming attack (...after a driver, high on PCP...) and pedestrian safety project were verified from news report: Goldstein, Joseph. "City Will Place 1,500 Bollards to Counter Vehicle Attacks." *The New York Times*, New York, 2 Jan. 2018, www.nytimes.com/2018/01/02/nyregion/city-will-place-1500-bollards-to-counter-vehicle-attacks.html. Accessed 28 Feb. 2026.

Details regarding a pedestrian safety project in London (London's Arsenal's Emirates Stadium...) were verified from news report: Halliday, Josh, and Perraudin, Frances. "What Can Be Done to Prevent Berlin-Style Attacks in Modern Cities," *The Guardian*, United States, 20 Dec. 2016, www.theguardian.com/uk-news/2016/dec/20/what-can-be-done-to-prevent-berlin-style-attacks-in-modern-cities. Accessed 28 Feb. 2026.

Details regarding a pedestrian safety project in Barcelona (...construction so-called "superblocks.") were verified from the following article: Roberts, David. "Cars Dominate Cities. Barcelona Has Set Out to Change That," *Vox*, 11 Sept. 2019, www.vox.com/energy-and-environment/2019/4/8/18273893/barcelona-spain-urban-planning-cars. Accessed 28 Feb. 2026. Also see "Effects on Health," www.barcelona.cat, ajuntament.barcelona.cat/qualitataire/en/la-salut/effects-health. Accessed 28 Feb. 2026.

Details of survivors' reactions (For Jenna...For Shamsi...) regarding Russell Weller's conviction are sourced in Chapter 2, "Victims, Survivors, Relive Horrors." Also see Chapter 43, "A New Sense of Loss at Farmers Market."

Details regarding what contributed (...pedal error and the lack of an adequate barrier system...) to the severity of the Farmers' Market crash are sourced in Prologue, NTSB. *Highway Accident Report*, "Analysis," p. 49

Descriptions of Russell Weller's character (...the man who coldly asked...) were verified from news report: Gold, Matea, et al. "Driver Involved in Crash Is Known for Helping Others." *SFGATE*, 17 July 2003, www.sfgate.com/news/article/driver-involved-in-crash-is-known-for-helping-2602193.php. Accessed 28 Feb. 2026. Also see Chapter 20, "Market Tragedy Took Driver's Spirit, Kin Say."

The quotes, "It would have meant a great deal to me...I'm sorry," were taken from the following news report: Barco, Mandalit del. "Jury Convicts Elderly California Driver of Manslaughter." *NPR*, 21 Nov. 2006, www.npr.org/2006/11/21/6517857/jury-convicts-elderly-california-driver-of-manslaughter. Accessed 28 Feb. 2026.

Details regarding an older driver (While being held in a detention center...) accident in Japan were verified from news report: "'What I Did Can Never Be Undone': Elderly Driver's Regret over Fatal Accident." *The Mainichi*, 20 May 2019, mainichi.jp/english/articles/20190520/p2a/00m/0na/014000c. Accessed 1 March 2026.

CHAPTER 51

The Quote, "I recall from the last time I saw Russell...," was taken from the following email exchange: Archer, Steven. Received by Melissa Cronin, Nov. 2009.

CHAPTER 53

Details regarding the background of Leroy Lattier (While researching the stories...) are sourced in Chapter 1, "Suddenly, They Were Gone."

Details regarding statements from Russell Weller *(What did Russell Weller say...?)* are sourced in Chapter 48, "Santa Monica Police Department Interview of George Russell Weller."

CHAPTER 55

All dialogue between George Russell Weller and police investigators is sourced in Chapter 48, "Santa Monica Police Department Interview of George Russell Weller."

Credits

Parts of this book first appeared, sometimes in slightly different form, in the following publications:

The Washington Post
The Jerusalem Post
USA Today
Narratively
Chicken Soup for the Soul (Recovering from Traumatic Brain Injuries; The Power of Forgiveness; Let It Go)
Brevity
About Place Journal
Tahoma Literary Review
Entropy
Purple Clover
Past Ten
Saranac Review
Under the Gum Tree
Humanthology
The Medical Literary Messenger
Preservation Foundation
Writerland
Hunger Mountain Journal

www.ingramcontent.com/pod-product-compliance
Lightning Source LLC
LaVergne TN
LVHW100850190926
848329LV00025B/199
9781955194563